Science Studies Yoga

A REVIEW OF PHYSIOLOGICAL DATA

by

James Funderburk, Ph.D.

WITH INTRODUCTION BY

BARBARA B. BROWN, Ph.D.

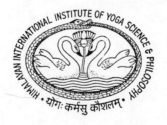

Published by

Himalayan International Institute
of Yoga Science & Philosophy of USA

ISBN: 0-89389-026-X

Copyright 1977

HIMALAYAN INTERNATIONAL INSTITUTE
OF YOGA SCIENCE & PHILOSOPHY OF USA

Great spirits have always encountered
violent opposition from mediocre minds.

Albert Einstein

Contents

Foreword

Yoga means union. It is a systematic approach to becoming one with, or attaining the highest level or state of consciousness of which man is capable. This attainment of his highest potential has been a perennial goal of mankind.

In order to unravel and dispel the obstacles that stood in the way of attaining the expanded consciousness and awareness that they sought, the yogic masters were forced over the ages to deal, one by one, with the different aspects of man's functioning. The functions of the body were systematically explored through a very precise series of postures or *asanas* which make up much of what is known today as "hatha yoga." Intricacies of respiration and breathing patterns were studied in great detail. The workings of the mind were catalogued and explained. This careful and precise approach to the functions of the mind and body established a series of clearly defined, easily reproducible, and, at the same time, beneficial practices which can profitably be studied in the modern laboratory. Over the last few decades the application of recent techniques for measuring physiological processes to the study of yoga, and statistical analysis of the results has produced a growing body of data. When it is brought together in a coherent form there emerges a picture of an impressive wealth of therapeutic techniques and research possibilities.

By bringing this information together, Dr. Funderburk has done a service to both the clinician and the research worker. The physician or the physical therapist who wishes to prescribe quiet, relaxing and yet effective methods of exercise is often attracted to the simplicity and calming effects of yogic practices. Now, with ready access to experimental data on the effects of these postures, exercises and meditation, the clinician can intelligently and effectively select the best assortment of practices for each individual patient. He need not guess. He can rely on solid, empirical data.

Yet much more data is needed. For this reason it is the research scientist who stands to benefit most from the information contained in *Science Studies Yoga*. Within these pages he can orient himself to what has been accomplished in the area of psychophysiological research into yoga and meditation. Up until this time it was almost impossible to do this because the data was so scattered. This collection of information, however, now permits the research worker to frame intelligent questions and know where his efforts will best be directed. Much work remains to be done.

For scientists who wish to explore the nature of the relationship between body and mind, a study of the effects of yoga postures, breathing exercises and meditation can be a virtual gold mine. Within these deceptively simple practices lie the fruits of thousands of years of careful and systematic exploration by a long line of sages. These dedicated men and women devoted their lives to the continuing perfection of a system of self-training (called *yoga*) that would bring the body and mind into harmony in such a way that man could realize his highest potential. Each of the techniques for body positioning, for breathing, for working with the mind, is designed, then, not only to contribute to health and personal evolution but to work synergistically with the other techniques. For this reason, within this spectrum of practices are the seeds of many therapeutic techniques, as well as, it seems likely, important and strategic clues to unravelling many of the mysteries of physiology and of the mind. It remains only for the research worker to take up, with the modern technological tools of the research laboratory, the study of these ancient and :imeless techniques. Thus we hope will continue the work that has already begun and which is so impressively outlined within the pages of this book.

Swami Rama
Himalayan Institute
Glenview, Illinois

Preface

For thousands of years individuals and small groups of individuals have systematically explored their own nature and that of the universe with the methods of yoga. On account of its systematic, experimental approach to personal growth, yoga has sometimes been referred to as a science. In the twentieth century the science of yoga has been the object of investigation by many scientists, representing physiology, medical research, and psychology. In the 1920's the first laboratory devoted to the study of yoga was established: Kaivalyadhama, at Lonavala, India. Along with the continuing systematic investigations of yoga at Kaivalyadhama, since the 1950's there have been studies on yoga and meditation by various university and research laboratories throughout the world. (See Appendix E for a list of investigators and laboratories.)

The purpose of this report is to summarize in some detail the physiological data that have emerged from scientific studies of yoga and meditation. Plausible inferences and explanatory conceptualizations have been shunned as premature. Instead, the extant data have been sifted, and data on similar physiological systems and variables (for example, the circulatory system and the heart rate) put together. Presentation of much of the data is given in graphical form (see Appendix B). Although hatha yoga and meditation together comprise the unified practice of yoga, most researchers have studied just one or the other and this separation between the two aspects of yoga that is found in the reported literature has guided our separation of this report into two parts:

Physiological Responses to Hatha Yoga (Part I)
Physiological Responses to Meditation (Part II)

This book is designed as an aid for further scientific study. It should be stressed that *all* available physiological data have been included, regardless of their positive or negative or neutral implications bearing on the possible benefits of yoga. Researchers will find a thorough overview of experimental results which, it is hoped, will stimulate more extensive investigations. Teachers and students of yoga will find a wealth of information that may be brought to their classes and practices for consideration. Medical doctors will find some data suggestive of therapeutic applications, although it should be noted that several purely clinical applications of yoga have not been explicitly dealt with in this account. That a small treatice such as this can give a glimpse of most facets of scientific research on yoga suggests the early and incomplete state of this art and the need for further intensive collaboration between mutually sympathetic scientists and yogis.

For complete understanding of the data reported, the reader will need some familiarity with yoga and with physiology. This background has been partially provided in the two glossaries, one of physiological terms and one of yogic terms. Texts such as those of Swami Rama (*Lectures on Yoga*)[1] and Swami Kuvalayananda (*Popular Yoga Asanas*)[2] are appropriate references to the concepts and practices of yoga. Any standard human physiology text would describe most physiological items mentioned.

Acknowledgements

The work of Sri Swami Rama, founder of the Himalayan International Institute of Yoga Science and Philosophy, in making yoga accessible to individuals with training in the sciences, has provided a climate where a treatise such as the present one is conceivable. Numerous factual corrections suggested by Swami Rama and O. P. Tiwari, Secretary of Kaivalyadhama (Lonavala, India), have been incorporated. Mark Siegchrist, of the English department of Marquette University, suggested ways in which the intended ideas of the book might be more clearly expressed. Any remaining inaccuracies and obscurities must be ascribed to the author, and he would welcome suggestions that readers may wish to communicate to him. The author also thanks his mother, Mrs. Doris Funderburk, for helpful assistance in the early stages of manuscript preparation, and the publication staff of the Himalayan Institute, particularly Theresa O'Brien and Janet Zima for excellent work in the final stages of the process of transforming the thought of this book into its present form.

James Funderburk
November, 1976

Introduction

After the first waves of Western interest in yogic practices, there has come the realization of the importance of yoga to the emotional and physical well-being of Western as well as of Eastern man. The 1970's have seen the development of a remarkable bonding between the mind-spirit approaches to health embodied in yoga and the physical approaches to health embraced by Western medicine.

It has not been an easy union. Less than twenty years ago the potential of yogic practices for ensuring well-being was disdained by American scientific authority. Yet today symposia, conferences, and courses on the usefulness of yoga to recover and maintain both mental and physical health can be found in the curricula of many of the most prominent American institutions serving the Health Sciences.

The reasons for the reversal in attitude are many. The expanding speed and depth of communications have provided us occidentals with an increasing understanding of the philosophic foundations of yoga and meditation. Jet travel and changing political attitudes have fostered the means for direct exchanges of information. Many Americans have been able to observe directly the yogic and meditation practices of India, while teachers and yoga masters from India have been able to establish important educational centers in the West. Another important factor contributing to the developing exchange of information and understanding has been the changing social psychologic interests and attitudes of the West. Almost as if preparing to receive new insights into the nature of man, the period of the 1960's in the United States was one of a growing restlessness and dissatisfaction with the prevailing philosophies, and a great distress for the condition of man in the midst of material plenty.

As the attention of the occidental became directed toward the potential of the mind, and growing numbers of people began to give testimony to the emotional and physical benefits of yoga and meditation, it became clear to science that there were meaningful new dimensions of medicine and psychotherapy to be explored. Neither medical science nor psychology had, in this century, formally acknowledged the role of mind and internal awarenesses in the healing process. With evidence available for the real benefits of yoga and meditation in healing, science now had to undertake confirmation of the evidence by the standards it had developed for the recognition of any health aid. This has meant, as is traditional in the scientific method, surveys and analyses of the existing literature, and new experimental work using the index of modern medicine and psychophysiology.

It was at this frontier of the new science of yoga and meditation that we owe a debt of gratitude to Dr. Funderburk. For most of us the scientific literature about yoga is difficult to obtain, and for many of us also the terminology is strange. In Dr. Funderburk's book the confusion of multi-faceted studies has been dispelled.

Many studies of the effects of yoga on physiologic systems either combine results for the different systems or differ in the aspects of yoga studied for a particular effect. The present review has systematically extracted the different elements of methodology and collated effects under the respective physiologic systems. Moreover, a large share of the data is presented in graphic form, allowing for rapid visual appreciation of results, and a glossary provides explanations for specialized yogic terminology.

Although Dr. Funderburk shies away from theoretical interpretations, the systematization of the data lets the results stand for themselves. The techniques and effectiveness of yoga and meditation can therefore be appreciated directly from what is accomplished, and the evidence is quantitative. I know of no other summary of yoga research that gives the data so objectively and in a form for such ready reference. The book doubtless will be of considerable importance to therapists and teachers alike, and should be most valuable in stimulating further research.

Dr. Barbara B. Brown
Veterans Administration Hospital
Sepulveda, California

Part I

Physiological Responses
to Hatha Yoga

·1·

Muscular~Articular
Responses to Hatha Yoga

A brief etymological reference indicates important distinctions between physical exercise and yoga *asanas*. *Exercise* is derived from *exercere*, a Latin word often regarded as having meant primarily to "drive forth (a tillage beast)" and hence "to employ, to set to work." In the context of physical exercise, *exercise* connotes exertion of the muscles and limbs. *Exertion* in turn means vigorous action, effort.

Asana, on the other hand, literally means *sitting position* or *posture*. As used by Patanjali, the codifier of Yoga science, *asana* refers to the attainment of a steady and comfortable posture for the practices of *pranayama* (control of *prana*), *pratyahara* (sense withdrawal) and *dhyana* (meditation). Thus, *asana* in this restrictive sense refers only to what may be called the meditative postures, which are varieties of sitting. Only later did the system of asanas evolve into the science of physical culture, into the system of postures playing a predominant role in hatha yoga.

The non-meditative asanas may be used to promote general physical well-being and are sometimes referred to as cultural asanas.

Those aphorisms in the *Yoga Sutras* of Patanjali which deal with asanas state that postures should be steady and comfortable. A posture is perfected (made steady and comfortable) not by forceful effort, but by relaxing and fixing the consciousness on the infinite. Though the *Yoga Sutras* are concerned explicitly with meditative postures, Patanjali nonetheless implicitly suggests the manner of practice of all the asanas as viewed by practitioners of Raja Yoga. Thus, in cultural asanas also, the emphasis is on stability, comfortableness and relaxation in the maintenance of a steady position.

A. EMG Studies

Objective assessment of muscular activity during standard physical exercise is usually a simple matter. One needs only to record the number of pounds lifted, the time in which a certain distance is run, etc. But such techniques are inappropriate for objectively assessing the degree of steadiness or relaxation attained in a yoga posture, and the more subtle technique of electromyography must be called upon as an appropriate measuring device. Electromyography is the method of measuring and recording the electrical activity coincidental with muscular activity. The degree of relaxation or contraction of a muscle is today defined in terms of electromyographic recordings (EMG). The EMG has been monitored during various yoga asanas.

A group of physical education teachers in India, who had performed yoga postures as a part of their training, was asked to spend a couple of weeks practicing every day, in their usual way, two particular asanas, the posterior stretching posture (*paschimottanasana*) and the half-spinal twist (*ardha-matsyendrasana*). The EMG activity was registered from back, buttock, thigh and calf muscles (specifically, from the *latissimus dorsi, gluteus maximus, biceps femoris* and *gastrocnemius*) during the performance of these postures. This was only half the experiment. Next, the subjects were instructed very specifically according to the precepts of Patanjali in the manner of practicing asanas. They were told to relax in the postures and to focus their thoughts on the infinite while in the postures in order to aid relaxation. After two weeks more of practicing the asanas, measurement of EMG activity was again registered. The major finding was that muscle activity, degree of excellence in the pose, and comfortable duration of holding the pose were all changed as a result of practicing the asanas according to the precepts of Patanjali. The degree of the strain of a muscle was classified by visual observation of the EMG as indicating either no activity of the muscle, negligible activity, slight activity, moderate activity, marked activity or very marked activity; these categories were assigned the integers 0 through 5, respectively. Average values for the before-minus-after differences of these numbers were calculated and tested for statistical significance. It was reported by P. V. Karambelkar[1] (see Figure 1.1) that average values of EMG activity were lower after practicing according to the instructions than before, for each muscle group and each asana. The improvement in relaxation of the buttock was significant (p < .01) for *paschimottanasana* (posterior-stretching posture) and *ardha-matsyendrasana* (half-spinal twist) on both right and left sides. Improvement of relaxation of the calf-muscle had a higher statistical significance (p < .01) for the posterior stretching posture than it had for the right and left half-spinal twist (p < .05). Relaxation of the thigh was statistically significant (p < .01) only for *paschimottanasana*. Relaxation of the back, though indicated, was not statistically significant for the postures. It was also seen in this experiment that duration of asana maintenance was in every subject increased from 10% to 50% by the mental adherence to relaxation and focus of attention on the infinite.

Investigations by K. S. Gopal[2] contrasted two groups of subjects: one group had been trained in asanas for a period of six months; the second group had no previous training in yoga but regularly engaged in light exercise. During the performance by both groups of a sequence of 8 asanas, various EMG recordings were obtained, and in each of the asanas the non-integrated EMG was greater for the untrained subjects than for the trained subjects. Training apparently made the performance of the asanas involve less muscular work. (See figure 1.2.) Among the asanas measured, it was stated that *shavasana* (corpse posture) required from each group the least muscular activity.

It should be noted that even the trained subjects in this experiment were not asserted to be experts in hatha yoga. It would be most desirable to have complete physiological portraits, including EMG, of expert practitioners of hatha yoga before, during and after the performance of various asanas. We hope this kind of study will be forthcoming in the near future.

Along the spinal column are three important cords. In the center is the *canalis centralis*, and on both sides lie the gangliated cords of the sympathetic nervous system. It is important that these three cords function in a normal and healthy way. With the help of the postures the spinal column remains supple and the spinal cords function in their normal manner. Allowing our spinal column to remain crooked creates discomfort while doing meditation. Health and strength of the abdominal musculature are needed to maintain the health of the intestinal track and to assist the diaphragm in breathing practices.

The first experiment discussed above showed that there was maintained tension in the back muscles in *paschimottanasana* (posterior stretching posture) and in *ardha-matsyendrasana* (half-spinal twist) even with the effort of relaxation. Indeed, half-spinal twist and so on, are designed especially to assure the strength of the musculature that maintains the integrity of the spinal curvature. The special practices called *bandhas*, or locks, especially require control of the abdominal musculature. X-ray studies have substantiated the prominent role of the *abdominal recti* muscles in the practice of *nauli.*[3]

B. Flexibility

It is found by those who practice yoga postures that an easily recognized benefit is increased flexibility.

V. Hubert Dhanaraj[4] measured a number of physiological variables and their changes after training either in yoga or in the 5BX Program for Physical Fitness. Fifty-one male college students, average age 18.8 years, were randomly assigned to a yoga training group, a 5BX training group, or a control group. The six weeks of training for the yoga group consisted of fifteen minutes of asanas —*bhujangasana* (cobra posture), *halasana* (plow posture), *sarvangasana* (shoulder stand), *matsyasana* (fish posture), and *shavasana* (corpse posture) and two minutes of pranayama. The six weeks of 5BX training consisted of eleven minutes for the 5BX standard graded sequence of exercises and four minutes of additional exercises. The control group received no exercise training and was instructed to maintain the usual level of physical activity. After the six weeks of training, the yoga group underwent a six weeks de-training period in which the subjects were instructed to forego yoga practices. Measurements were made before and after each six week period.

Dhanaraj[4] found that after only six weeks of daily practice of the yoga routine, there was an increase in a measure of flexibility. (The Wells Sit-and-Reach Test; see Figure 1.3.) The group which practiced the 5BX Program for Physical Fitness also showed a flexibility increase, although of lesser magnitude than that of the yoga group. The difference between pre-training and post-training scores was statistically highly significant ($p < .005$) for both groups, as was the difference between the improvement in flexibility of the two groups. The post-detraining decrease in flexibility for the yoga group was statistically significant.

Robson Moses[5] considered changes in flexibility (extension-flexion ranges) of the left ankle, the hip, the hip and trunk combined, and the neck. Experimental and control groups, each composed of 27 male subjects, were chosen at random from physical education classes at a university. Measurements were made before and after ten weeks of a hatha yoga class for the experimental group, and before and after ten weeks in various physical education classes for the control group. Postures taught in the yoga course included *halasana* (plough posture), *sarvangasana* (shoulder stand), *bhujangasana* (cobra posture), *shalabhasana* (locust posture), *chakrasana* (wheel posture), *matsyasana* (fish posture), *yoga mudra* (symbol of yoga), *simhasana* (lion posture), *padmasana* (lotus posture), and *shavasana* (corpse posture). Breathing exercises taught in the yoga course included *ujjayi* (for definition, see Appendix D), *nadi shodhana* (alternate nostril breathing), *shitali* (cooling breath), and *bhastrika* (bellows). Statistical analysis of the measurements showed significant increases in flexibility for the yoga group as compared with the control group for hip, hip and trunk, and neck, although not for ankle. (See Figure 1.4.)

Hatha yoga practices, of course, are not designed to increase the fitness of the individual as measured by certain traditional tests. Nevertheless, after administering several tests of physical fitness before and after a three-week program of yoga training, M. L. Gharote[6] found the scores of such tests to increase. The yoga training followed the recommendations of a National Plan for Physical Education of the Government of India's Ministry of Education. It included training in twenty asanas, three *kriyas (agnisara, kapalabhati [nauli], and nauli), uddiyana-bandha* (abdominal lock), and *ujjayi pranayama* without retention; the training for women did not include *mayurasana* (peacock posture). Males were given tests to measure the following fitness factors: extent flexibility, dynamic flexibility, explosive strength, dynamic strength, trunk strength, coordination, equilibrium, and stamina. Females were given tests to measure the fitness factors of extent flexibility, dynamic flexibility, trunk strength and equilibrium. When test scores were converted into an overall fitness index, Gharote found that the three weeks of yoga practice caused statistically significant (p < .01) positive changes in the fitness index for both males and females. (See Figure 1.5.)

C. Pressure Changes in Internal Cavities

At this point, we turn to a consideration of *bandhas*, or locks, in yoga. These locks involve control of the diaphragm and the anal sphincters. The *bandhas* are sometimes accessories to the practice of pranayama and may be viewed as methods of controlling the distribution of energy within the body. We will primarily consider *uddiyana-bandha* (abdominal lock) and certain of its variations. The basic idea of *uddiyana-bandha* is to exhale completely and then make a mock inhalation; that is, make an inhalatory thoracic movement but at the same time close the glottis so the air does not enter the chest. It has been shown in X-ray studies conducted by Swami Kuvalayananda[7] that the diaphragm rises to a greater extent during application of *uddiyana-bandha* than in a normal expiration. Also, the colon is raised so that relative to the vertebral column it is higher than normal and its transverse portion may even be curved upward in some individuals. In addition to the change in position of the diaphragm, which decreases the vertical capacity of the thorax, there is a lateral movement of the ribs which increases the horizontal, or lateral, thoracic capacity. When *uddiyana-bandha* is applied, the abdomen is pulled in to a great extent even without voluntary effort of the abdominal muscles. When *nauli* is performed, this movement of the abdomen is reversed, and control is exerted over another one or both of the abdominal recti so that a portion of the abdominal wall accordingly is extended.

Uddiyana-bandha (abdominal lock) and its extensions of *nauli* (central, right and left) have been shown to produce sub-atmospheric pressure of considerable magnitude in the various internal cavities. These sub-atmospheric pressures were first noted by Swami Kuvalayananda[8] in a sequence of experiments in the 1920's and have later been confirmed by other studies[9] in the Kaivalyadhama laboratories.   (See Figure 1.6.)   The absolute values of the sub-atmospheric pressures within the esophagus, stomach, colon and bladder are least in *uddiyana-bandha*, intermediate in right and left *nauli*, and greatest in central *nauli*. These pressures are more extreme than the negative pressures normally occurring during inspiration. During *uddiyana-bandha*, esophageal and intragastric pressures are more negative than colonic and bladder pressures.   In *nauli*, the magnitude of esophageal pressure is least and that of gastric pressure greatest, whereas colonic pressures are intermediate.

The data just discussed were obtained by directly measuring the air pressure in the various internal cavities. Other experiments have indirectly confirmed that data. M. A. Wenger [10] observed that with a catheter certain practitioners of yoga could, for the purpose of cleansing, draw water into the bladder or the colon. This phenomenon was examined in experiments by M. V. Bhole,[11] where the amount and rate of water drawn into the stomach, bladder and colon were recorded during *uddiyana-bandha* (abdominal lock) and *nauli*. (See Figures 1.7 and 1.8.) The motion of water into these cavities when *nauli* or *uddiyana-bandha* was performed indicates that the pressure within the cavities was less than the pressure on the water outside. It was found that during both *uddiyana-bandha* and *nauli* the volume and rate of water suction were greater into the stomach than into either the bladder or the colon. This finding is consistent with the greater negativity of pressure in the stomach than in the bladder or colon. (See Figure 1.6.) No water was drawn into the colon during *uddiyana-bandha*. During *nauli* the volume and rate of water drawn into the colon were greater than the volume and rate of water drawn into the bladder. This relation is inconsistent with the greater extremity of bladder pressure in comparison to colonic pressure, but may be explained by size differences between the urinary passageway and the colon. Finally, volume and rate of water suction were less in *uddiyana-bandha* than *nauli*, consistent with the greater pressure applied during *nauli*.

Swami Kuvalayananda[12] explained the sub-atmospheric pressures during *uddiyana-bandha* and its variations in part as follows. The greatly raised diaphragm has two effects: 1) it lowers the pressure of gases in the abdominal cavity, thereby leading to involuntary inward abdominal motion as a result of the greater atmospheric pressure external to the abdomen; 2) it tends to decrease thoracic volume, thereby increasing thoracic pressure. Now, sub-atmospheric intra-esophageal pressures imply sub-atmospheric intra-thoracic pressures, since the esophagus is within the thorax. Thus, the tendency toward decreased thoracic volume mentioned in 2) above is somehow overcome during *uddiyana-bandha*. Apparently lateral thoracic expansion by upward rib movement is greater than vertical thoracic diminution by upward diaphragmatic movement. In short, thoracic volume increases during *uddiyana-banda*; since the closed glottis prohibits further air entry into the lungs, the intra-thoracic pressure is lessened. Intra-esophageal pressures are less negative than intra-gastric pressures because of rigidity of the cartilaginous esophageal rings and distensibility of the stomach. The fact that the pressures, especially in the stomach, are more extreme during *nauli* than during *uddiyana-bandha* may be due to increased abdominal size occasioned by the outward motion of the abdominal wall. The slightly greater magnitude of sub-atmospheric pressures in the esophagus during *nauli* may be explained by the communication of the esophageal cavity with that of the stomach.

One other aspect of *uddiyana-bandha* may be mentioned. X-ray analysis[13] showed a change in distribution of colonic contents as well as a change in colonic position. The ascending and descending colon were shifted upward and their lower aspects were pulled toward the vertebral column. The transverse colon shifted from sagging downward to arching upward. Colonic contents were focussed in the transverse colon with minimal amounts in the ascending and descending colons.

Sub-atmospheric internal pressures have also been recorded in *agnisara*. In the practice of *agnisara*, the breath is retained after deep exhalation, while the abdomen is alternately retracted and protracted; each retraction and protraction is maintained for a few seconds, and the process is continued until another breath is needed. Intra-gastric pressure changes during *agnisara* have been reported as follows.[14] Slightly positive (15-20 mm. Hg.) intra-gastric pressure was noted during the deep expiration preliminary to *agnisara*. This positive pressure went to zero with the retraction of the abdominal wall during *agnisara*. When the abdominal wall was protracted, highly negative (-110 to -120 mm. Hg.) intra-gastric pressure occurred initially, but during the maintenance of the abdominal protraction the pressures soon fell to a steady value, between -50 and -60 mm. Hg.

Positive intra-gastric pressures have also been noted[15] during the performance of several asanas. (See Figure 1.9.) The average intra-gastric pressures for several subjects were largest during *mayurasana* (peacock posture) and *shalabhasana* (locust posture) —72.5 mm. Hg. and 65.5 mm. Hg. respectively; the most extreme reading was 100 mm. Hg. for one subject during *shalabhasana*.

D. The Power of Breath

In considering remarkable feats in the realm of physical activity, scientific investigators, even more than the general public, may be interested in trying to fathom the method by which such feats are performed. Individuals trained in yoga have been observed, by men trained in the methods of science to observe impartially, to perform various such feats. This study will here describe reports of certain demonstrations given by one subject, Yogi Ramananda of Mysore. Yogi Ramananda is a 106 pound,

67 year-old (in 1976) male citizen of India, who has been practicing yoga since the age of 30. At the age of 48 he participated in a confinement experiment conducted by H. V. G. Rao, at the All-India Institute of Mental Health in Bangalore, results of which are described elsewhere in this book (see Chapter 2, Section C). He has also been involved in experiments conducted at the Kaivalyadhama laboratories in Lonavala, India. In June of 1976 he was a participant in the International Yoga and Meditation Conference held in Chicago under the auspices of the Himalayan International Institute of Yoga Science and Philosophy. As a result of this Conference, Yogi Ramananda was studied by the Himalayan Institute and Forest Hospital, Des Plaines, Illinois, under the general direction of Rudolph M. Ballentine, Jr., M.D. and the technical assistance of Robert Gibbons. These experiments included physiological monitoring of Yogi Ramananda during a confinement period and during his demonstration of two unusual feats of strength. These latter events we now describe.

Rao[16] had noted that Yogi Ramananda "could use his bare fingers (first and middle) like a pair of scissors to cut a leaf into two. He claimed that he was able to do this by concentrating all his energy on his fingers." Gibbons observed the same phenomenon; a rolled leaf would be severed in such a manner that one piece would be propelled several feet away.

Rao also noted that the subject "was able to break a chain into two by winding it around the waist and extending it with the foot. One could see the chain, which was made of 3/8 inch iron bar, gradually give way to the pressure." Ballentine and Gibbons[17] provided a more detailed description of his observations of the chain breaking. Preliminary to the demonstration, the subject underwent a full test of physical strength conducted by the Occupational Therapy Department of another nearby hospital. This test showed the subject's physical strength to be normal for his age group. Next, the chain to be broken was tested, and shown to require a tension of 650 pounds before a link began to bend. During the period of breaking the chain the subject was monitored both by video tape and by a gas analyzer which was set up to analyze each breath the subject took. The chain was then wrapped around the subject's waist and connected back to itself, leaving nine single links in front of the subject. The ninth link was connected to a metal bar on which the subject placed his feet, causing tension in the nine links. After the subject's normal respiration was measured for 2 minutes, he was given the signal to break the chain. The 2-minute period showed a respiratory rate of 6 breaths per minute. When asked to break the chain, the subject was measured to increase the respiratory rate to 18 breaths per minute for a duration of one minute. Then he took one breath (O_2 analyzed at 21%) for 13 seconds and exhaled at the time of the chain's breakage. Upon examination the link that broke was found to be severed in half, rather than bent open.

·2·

Circulatory Responses
to Hatha Yoga

Our discussion of the effects of asanas on the skeletal-muscular system has suggested that the purpose of asanas has nothing to do with development of muscularity. Rather, they are intended to prepare the body internally for the practice of meditation, as is well exemplified in the following discussion of the effects of hatha yoga on the circulatory system. In view of the breadth and subtlety of such effects one can only wonder at the level of sophistication in knowledge of human physiology that gave birth to the development of the system of asanas. Further, in view of the wide range of benefits from the supplementary phases of hatha yoga in the system of Raja Yoga, one begins to glimpse the profundity of the system of Raja Yoga.

After a preliminary statement of the effect of hatha yoga on the circulatory system, we will consider its effects on blood flow alterations, heart activity, blood pressure and blood contents.

A. Cardiovascular Efficiency

Just as a program of yoga practices has been shown to increase a cumulative index of physical fitness (see Figure 1.5), so also has such a program been measured to have an overall effect on cardiovascular efficiency, even though yoga practices are not explicitly intended to affect the factors measured by these tests. Cardiovascular efficiency denotes the capacity of an individual to maintain strenuous activity of the whole body for a prolonged period.

An index widely used to determine overall cardiovascular efficiency is the Harvard Step Test. The Harvard Step Test requires a subject to step up and down on a bench rhythmically over a 5-minute period or until he cannot maintain the correct performance due to fatigue. Shortly afterwards the pulse is measured for half-minute intervals. The total time of correct performance of the stepping and the number of pulse counts are noted, and a ratio of the duration of the exercise by the number of pulse counts gives the score for the Harvard Step Test. This test has been used for, among other things, selecting men for hard physical labor. Higher scores indicate greater cardiovascular efficiency.

Ganguly[1] measured scores on the Harvard Step Test in a study involving 11 clinically normal males of average age 26 years. The subjects were measured before and after 8 months of yoga training, which consisted of one hour yoga practice daily including asanas, *kriyas* (cleansing practices), pranayamas, *bandhas* (locks), *mudras* (seals) and meditation. There was found to be an average increase of 7.6 in the test score, from 78.6 to 86.2; this was a statistically significant change ($p < .05$). (See Figure 2.1.) One of the 5 subjects initially scoring in the high average category (65-79) remained in that category, while 3 moved to the good category (80-89) and 1 to the excellent (90 and above) category. Four of the 6 subjects initially in the good category remained in that category after testing, while 2 moved to the excellent category. (See Figure 2.2.)

It is perhaps paradoxical that a program of yoga practices, which do not involve vigorous exercises, has been seen to promote cardiovascular efficiency. To date, no comparisons in a controlled setting have been made between yoga practices as opposed to programs of vigorous exercise in terms of promoting cardiovascular efficiency. Also of interest would be the determination of which aspects of yoga account for this effect. We now turn to some more detailed studies whose analysis by researchers may suggest how this effect may come about. (Since Harvard Step Test scores are indicative of maximal oxygen intake in exercise, certain aspects of the next chapter of this book, on respiratory effects of hatha yoga, are also relevant.)

Blood Flow Alterations

Although a simple model of the circulatory system is that of a system of closed tubing through which a fluid is propelled by means of a pump, one very great modification of this model is that the diameter of various parts of this tubing can change for various reasons. These changes in blood vessel diameter permit variations in blood supply to different regions. If an organ or system is active, then it receives a greater blood flow. Application of this principle leads to some inferences regarding blood flow alterations in asanas. Most articular regions receive increased blood flow for a period of time during a practice session of asanas, as nearly every joint is put through its range of motion. Asanas especially involve limbering the vertebral joints through forward, backward and lateral bends in the cervical through sacral regions. The activity of neck, back, chest and abdominal muscles accompanies the various trunk movements. In *mayurasana* (peacock posture), pressure of the elbows on the abdomen may result in increased blood flow to certain internal abdominal organs, such as the pancreas. Most asanas do not require exertion of, and consequently do not divert large blood supplies to, the major muscles of the limbs.

To a casual observer of someone performing asanas, the inverted postures, such as *sarvangasana* (shoulder stand) and *shirshasana* (headstand), are particularly remarkable. We will now consider the effects such postures may have on the blood flow. Since the veins which return the de-oxygenated blood to the heart usually have thin distensible walls and since there is very little pressure in the venous blood to push it forward, the question arises as to how the blood travels through the veins and arrives at the heart. Ordinarily, this is accomplished in part by muscular movements which rhythmically squeeze the veins and, since the veins contain one-way valves, propel the blood toward the heart. Common experience suggests that inadequate muscular activity, during prolonged standing or sitting, leads to congestion of blood in the lower parts of the body. The condition of varicose veins may be one outcome of a long occurrence of this phenomenon. The inverted postures re-arrange the body parts so that gravity, instead of opposing, assists in the drainage of blood from the lower limbs and trunk.

In *sarvangasana* (shoulder stand), not only is the flow of venous blood from the lower extremities of the body to the heart accentuated, but also there is an increase of blood flow to the neck, including the region of the thyroid gland. This latter effect is due in part to gravitational forces focussing on the neck which is the lowest body point during *sarvangasana*, and in part to the pressure in the thyroid region due to the firm placement of the chin in the jugular notch. We will see evidence supportive of these assertions in later examinations of blood pressure readings in the various asanas. Since the thyroid gland is highly vascular, diversion of blood flow to the neck region is helpful in maintaining the health of this gland, whose outputs are important to the general metabolic activities of the body. *Shirshasana* (headstand) has most of the same effects of venous drainage as *sarvangasana* (shoulder stand), but differs in that the lowest point is the head.

S. Rao[2] has compared various cardiovascular responses

occurring in horizontal supine position, erect standing position and headstand posture. The subjects, six male medical school students, had some experience with the headstand posture and could maintain it for up to fifteen minutes. Measurements in the headstand posture were recorded after about five minutes had elapsed in the posture, to help assure that the readings were taken with the subject in stable state. In part of this study the average blood flow in a toe and a finger were determined by plethysmography. It was found (see Figure 2.3) that blood flow in the toe was less and blood flow in the finger was greater during the headstand than during either the horizontal supine position or the erect standing position. The average value for the blood flow in the toe was greater than that for the finger in the supine and erect positions but slightly less than that for the finger in the headstand posture. Rao also measured the forehead temperature and the top-of-the-foot skin temperature. The forehead skin temperature increased and the skin temperature of the dorsum of the foot decreased during the headstand as compared to other body positions. (See Figure 2.4.)

Gopal and Wenger have both presented data concerning finger blood flow in various practices of hatha yoga. Gopal's measurements were of two groups, each with fourteen male subjects; one group had been trained in asanas and pranayamas for at least six months while the other group had no yoga training but took long walks and played light games regularly. Wenger's data are from yoga students who had practiced yoga regularly for more than two years in the ashram at Kaivalyadhama, Lonavala, India.

In one part of his studies Gopal[3] reports finger blood flow, as measured plethysmographically, for both groups during performance of a sequence of seven yoga practices. (See Figure 2.5.) For the untrained subjects finger blood flow was least in *viparitakarani* (inverted action), *sarvangasana* (shoulder stand), and *shirshasana* (headstand), and was greatest in *dharmicasana* (symbol of yoga) and *shavasana* (corpse posture). For the trained subjects, finger blood flow was least in the headstand and greatest in *dharmicasana*, although almost as great in *shavasana*.

That finger blood flow was less among Gopal's subjects in the headstand than in *shavasana* (in which the body is in a horizontal supine position) appears to differ from the results of Rao described above. A tentative resolution of the apparent difference may be found in the recognition of the conscious relaxation, mental and physical, that the practitioner of *shavasana* undergoes. This relaxation could lessen the constriction of blood vessels in the periphery of the body, thereby increasing peripheral blood flow. The horizontal supine position, without the conscious relaxation, could be expected to have less effect on vasodilation of peripheral blood vessels.

Indeed, Gopal interprets the maximality of blood flow in *shavasana* as indicative of the relaxation of the subjects in this posture. He also interprets, as indicative of decreased autonomic nervous system activity, the fact that those subjects trained in yoga showed greater peripheral blood flow, in each position, than did those who were untrained.

Gopal[4] also measured peripheral blood flow as his two groups of subjects practiced various breathing patterns with and without application of *bandhas* (locks). (See Figure 2.6.) For both groups finger blood flow was less in inspiratory phases (inspiration-retention, deep inspiration with and without application of *bandhas*) than in expiratory phases; the value was least in deep inspiration with the *bandhas* and greatest in deep expiration without the *bandhas*. The peripheral blood flow was again less in all cases for untrained subjects than for trained subjects. The similar shape of the two curves in each of Figures 2.5 and 2.6 suggests that the effects of the various practices are similar in both groups of subjects, although they are more pronounced in the trained subjects.

Wenger[5] found little change either in finger temperature

or in finger pulse volume as his subjects practiced *shavasana* (corpse posture). (See Figures 5.1 and 5.2.) Wenger also measured finger temperature and finger pulse volume before, during and after the breathing practices of *ujjayi, bhastrika* (bellows), hyperventilation after *bhastrika, kapalabhati* (skull shining) and hyperventilation after *kapalabhati*. (See Figures 2.7, 2.8, 2.9, 2.10.) In all cases the average finger temperature decreased during the exercise period and the decrease was slightly greater in the pranayama exercises than in the non-yogic practice of hyperventilation. Finger pulse volume decreased during all practices except *kapalabhati*, during which it increased. The post-exercise finger pulse volumes returned to the pre-exercise level or higher after the *pranayama* exercises, but remained lower than the pre-exercise level when measured shortly after hyperventilation. Finger pulse volume was highest in the practice of *kapalabhati*, next in *ujjayi*, next in *bhastrika*, and lowest in hyperventilation.

In this discussion of the control of blood flow, we may mention the high degree of control over blood flow that has been demonstrated by a yogi in a study at the Menninger Foundation.[6] Thermistors were attached to the thenar and hypothenar imminences of the right hand of Swami Rama, who was providing the demonstration. In a matter of a few minutes there was produced a temperature difference of 10 degrees Celsius between the two electrodes: thenar temperature decreased and hypothenar temperature increased. The experimenters observed that this was not accomplished by any overt action of the skeletal musculature. They did observe, however, that the breathing pattern changed, in that the breath rate decreased. It has recently been suggested that tumor control might be possible if blood flow to the tumor region could be restricted: the great degree of vascularization involved in and necessary for the growth of tumors would thus be abated.

C. Heart Rate

The amount of blood pumped per unit time by the heart through the circulatory system depends on the number of contractions, or beats, of the heart in a given time interval and on the volume of blood propelled by the heart in a given contraction. Of course, the heart rate varies in response to a great many different factors; for example, it is higher during physical exertion or mental disquietude than it is during a restful state. Thus, the state in which heart rate is measured must be specified. We will here consider the effect of yoga training and practices on heart rate and the phenomenon of control of heart activity.

Dhanaraj[7] found that after 6 weeks of training, both a yoga group and a 5BX group demonstrated decreases in the heart rate in basal state by a small (3 to 4 beats/minute) but statistically significant ($p < .05$) amount. There was no appreciable change in a control group. (See Figure 2.11.)

Gopal[8] reported that subjects who were trained for 6 months in yoga demonstrated a lower heart rate during the performance of a variety of yoga practices than did those who performed the practices without previous training. (See Figures 2.12 and 2.13.)

In 2 studies K. N. Udupa and his colleagues considered various physiological effects of yoga practices. In the first study[9] 12 males, average age 23 years, underwent a systematic training in various hatha yoga practices. The daily one-hour training sessions continued for 6 months.

Yoga practices that were progressively introduced to subjects included the following: *bhujangasana* (cobra posture), *ardha-halasana* (half-plough posture), *eka-pada hastasana* (head-knee posture), *vakrasana* (twisted posture), *chakrasana* (wheel posture), *padmasana* (lotus posture), *halasana* (plough posture), *paschimottanasana* (posterior stretching posture), *shalabhasana* (locust posture), *viparitakarani* (inverted action), *simha-mudra* (symbol of the lion), *dhanurasana* (bow posture), *supta vajrasana* (supine pelvic posture), *ardha-matsyendrasana* (half-spinal twist), *yoga mudra* (symbol of yoga), *sarvangasana* (shoulder stand), *kapalabhati* (skull shining), *shirshasana* (headstand), *mayurasana* (peacock posture), *matsyasana* (fish posture), *kukkutasana* (cock posture), *garbhasana* (child-in-womb posture), *neti jala* (nostril cleansing with water), *neti sutra* (nostril cleansing with string), *ujjayi, bhastrika* (bellows), *uddiyana-bandha* (abdominal lock), *nauli.* Measurements were reported initially and after 3 and 6 months of training. In the second study [10] only four subjects, average age 20 years, were considered, and the practices involved lasted for three months. Two subjects practiced *surya-namaskar* (sun salutation) seven minutes a day. *Suryanamaskar* is not considered to be in the group of yogic practices; it is considered as a preliminary to hatha yoga, to make the body supple. One subject practiced *shirshasana* (headstand) seven minutes daily and *mayurasana* (peacock posture) three minutes daily; one subject practiced *sarvangasana* (shoulder stand) nine minutes, *matsyasana* (fish posture) two minutes and *halasana* (plough posture) three minutes, all on a daily basis. Measurements were noted before and after the three months of practice.

After three months of hatha yoga practices by the 12 subjects, average pulse rate in resting state was found by Udupa[11] to have decreased somewhat; this lower level was maintained after three more months of practice. (See Figure 2.14.) The amount by which the pulse rate increased in response to the physical stress of fast running was, after 6 months practice of yoga by Udupa's 12 subjects, less than initially; the difference between these values was not statistically significant, however. (See Figure 2.15.)

In the second study [12] of four subjects, after three months of practice of *suryanamaskar* (sun salutation) the pulse rate in standing position decreased by about 8 per minute for two of Udupa's subjects; pulse rate in sitting position changed very little. The pulse rate, in standing or sitting position, changed very little for a subject who practiced *shirshasana* (headstand) and *mayurasana* (peacock posture). After three months of practice of *sarvangasana* (shoulder stand), *matsyasana* (fish posture) and *halasana* (plow posture) the pulse rate of one subject decreased in both standing (6 per minute) and sitting (5 per minute). (See Figure 2.16.)

The direction of heart rate change, whether an increase or decrease, in response to various asanas and breathing practices was found by Gopal to be similar for subjects whether or not they were trained in hatha yoga.[13] (See Figures 2.12 and 2.13.) For both a trained and untrained group, heart rate was greatest in the practice of *setubandhasana* (bridge posture). In several breathing practices, heart rate was greatest for both groups during a deep inspiration with *bandhas* (locks); it was least for the trained group in deep expiration without the *bandhas* and least for the untrained group in rhythmic expiration-retention.

In the practice of yoga breathing exercises and of hyperventilation by yoga students, average heart rate was measured by Wenger[14] to be higher than the pre-exercise level. The elevation was 2 beats per minute during *bhastrika* (bellows), 4 during *ujjayi* and 12 during *kapalabhati* (skull shining.) The elevations were much greater in hyperventilation, amounting to increases of 28 to 32 beats per minute. (See Figures 2.17 and 2.18.)

Heart rate has been seen to increase during the practice of *sarvangasana* (shoulder stand) by about 60% over its basal state.[15] (See Figure 2.19.) In going from horizontal supine position to an erect standing position, subjects experienced[16] an average heart rate increase from 67 to 84; (see Figure 2.20) when *shirshasana* (headstand) was assumed it decreased to 69; after resumption of horizontal supine position subsequent to headstand, the average heart rate decreased to 63, below its initial value in the same position.

Fifteen minutes of practice of *shavasana* (corpse posture) lowered the heart rate an average of about 10 beats per minute. The same amount of time of simple rest in supine position lowered the heart rate by 4 beats per minute. This difference of 6 beats per minute was reported by Dhanaraj[17] to be not statistically significant. (See Figure 5.3.) Wenger [18] found little difference between heart rate measurements recorded before and during *shavasana* relaxation. (See Figure 5.4.)

Experiments have been designed to determine whether yoga practices have an effect on the heart's activity during and after physical exertion. PWC_{130} and PWC_{170} scores were obtained by Dhanaraj[19] before and after 6 weeks for a group trained in yoga, a group trained in the 5BX Program and a control group. (See Figure 2.21 and 2.22.) PWC is an abbreviation for physical work capacity. PWC_{130} is the intensity of work, or work per unit time, that a subject can perform when his heart rate is 130 beats per minute. A higher value of physical work capacity at a given heart rate suggests a greater work capability at that level of heart exertion. PWC_{170} gives the work capacity at a strenuous level of heart activity, PWC_{130} at a less strenuous but still vigorous level. The differences between pre-training and post-training in physical work capacity were in the direction of increased capacity for both the yoga group and the 5BX group; these differences were statistically significant at both heart rate levels for the 5BX group and at the lower (130) heart rate level for the yoga group; little change was seen in the control group scores.

In the same study, maximal heart rate showed a nonsignificant decrease after 6 weeks of yoga training. (See Figure 2.23.)

It may be recalled (see Figure 2.1) that a program of yoga practices increased a ratio of pulse count after exercise divided by amount of exercise. Such a result could be attributed to enhanced ability at pulse deceleration. There is some data available relevant to this question. A mean heart rate of about 71 beats per minute was found by Gopal[20] for a group which had been trained in yoga for 6 months and for a group which regularly engaged in long walks and light games. Afterwards both groups did twenty jumps and twenty sit-ups; the yoga group's mean heart rate increased to 100, about 7 less than that of the light exercise group. (See Figure 2.24.) A group with at least 6 weeks of certain hatha yoga practices followed strenuous exercise with 1 minute of sitting and then 3 minutes of either sitting, mild exercise, or *shavasana* (corpse posture) relaxation.[21] Just after the exercise, heart rate averaged over 180, and after 1 minute of sitting it had dropped to about 130. After 3 more minutes of sitting, (see Figure 2.25) it had dropped 17 more beats per minute, a lesser drop than that (22) following 3 minutes of mild exercise or than that (29) following 3 minutes of *shavasana* relaxation. This suggests that *shavasana* relaxation facilitates pulse deceleration following exercise. The investigator, Dhanaraj,[22] also found that, after five minutes of sitting, heart rate decreased more when *shavasana* relaxation was practiced by those trained for 6 weeks in yoga than it did when the same subjects before the training, or subjects in a control group, rested in supine position. (See Figure 2.26.)

There have been several studies of individuals during and after their confinement in more or less air-tight compartments. Studies of such pit "burials," as they are sometimes referred to, have been suggested to researchers from reports of cessation or reduction in biological functioning by yogis. For example, in nineteenth-century India, a yogi is said to have been buried for several months in a steel box; after this period of time he came out safely. Major goals of scientific studies have been to determine (a) if given individuals with experience in yoga show characteristic bodily functioning in such closed environments, and (b) how changes manifested by such individuals compare with changes in less trained or untrained persons placed in similar environments.

The electrocardiogram (ECG) of various subjects in confinement studies has been recorded. H. V. G. Rao[23] studied Yogi Ramananda of Mysore during 3 confinement periods, lasting 2, 9 and 8½ hours, in a pit of dimensions 2½' x 3' x 4'. Among the various types of physiological measurements obtained by Rao were ECG and spirogram. The ECG showed a steady heart beat throughout with a regular pattern of electrical activity. The heart rate varied within the limits of 40 and 100 beats per minute. Some slow and irregular heart rate variations were noted to parallel roughly similar changes in the spirogram.

Ballentine and Gibbons[24] have recently collected data from this same subject, Yogi Ramananda of Mysore, in a confinement experiment. An oxygen tent was modified into an air-tight compartment in which the subject sat. Before sealing the tent, leads for monitoring EEG, ECG, and EMG were connected to the subject. A lead was placed near the subject's nostrils for gas analysis. The gas analyzer used (MGA-series 1100, Perkin-Elmer Corporation) was capable of monitoring nitrogen, oxygen and carbon dioxide directly from the closed environment and recording percentages of each continuously. Full monitoring of all scales, including respiratory rate, continued throughout the experiment until the subject found the environment unbearable and requested the experiment's termination. Two hours before and 3 minutes after the confinement blood (venous) was drawn and a full blood gas analysis was conducted on both samples.

The subject signaled to be released after 33.0 minutes of confinement. Up through 31.5 minutes of confinement the ECG was normal. The venous blood gas analyses showed increases in carbon dioxide (25 to 33 milliequivalents/liter), the partial pressure of carbon dioxide (50 to 55 mm. Hg.), pH (7.29 to 7.38) and acid/base (14/-3 to 17/6 mm. Hg.) It showed decreases in the partial pressure of oxygen (38 to 29 mm. Hg.) and oxygen saturation (67% to 56%). Except for the high

acid/base values both before and after the confinement, all
values were within or close to normative data. Results of the
other data obtained by Gibbons are reported in appropriate
sections elsewhere in this book.

B. K. Anand[25] studied an individual (Yogi Ramananda of
Andhra) experienced in yoga who had asserted his previous
experience in prolonged sealed underground pit environments.
Prior to going into the closed environment, the subject's heart
rate was about 85 beats per minute. After half an hour of
confinement the heart rate had decreased and remained in the
range of 60 to 72 until about an hour before the end of the confinement; during the last hour the heart rate rose to about 80.
No ECG abnormalities were noted in the two confinement
trials, one lasting 8 hours and one 10 hours. About 2 hours
after the termination of confinement, the subject's body temperature rose to 101.5° F; this body temperature persisted
for about 6 hours and was reported by the subject to be a normal
feature of post-confinement periods.

In a study of several subjects undertaken by Karambelkar[26] it was found that the heart rate remained essentially
constant until the rate level of carbon dioxide content of the
pit reached 5% at which time the heart rate increased greatly;
the heart rate increased by about 50% over the constant level
when the carbon dioxide concentration reached 7%. In comparing those subjects who had practiced yoga and those who had
not, Karambelkar concluded that the increased heart rate did
not depend upon the amount of practice of yoga but rather
related to the concentration of carbon dioxide in the pit.

D. Heart Control

Next, we consider the results that have been found relative
to the phenomenon of heart control. It is a fact that some
individuals in India have been able to control their heart rhythm

even to the extent of stopping it.

The act of voluntarily stopping the heart from pumping blood is such an extraordinary phenomenon that it has aroused the interest of a number of scientific investigators. An early (1936) article by Brosse[27] reported affirmatively on the control by yogis of heart rate. The subjects for this study were described as both Hatha Yogis and Raja Yogis; the most significant results obtained were from the Hatha Yogis. The records presented consist of simultaneous pulse, respiration and electrocardiogram measurements made over a period of 2 months of experiments with various subjects. The results discussed occurred when the subjects were practicing some form of breath control and/or concentration. The phases of practicing control of the heart usually occurred during periods of apnea, either with full or empty lungs. Such periods either involved absolute cessation of breathing or very superficial respiration. Usually, tension of the respiratory muscles accompanied efforts of forced respiration in the first part of the period of apnea. The greatest changes in the electrocardiogram were during the relaxed periods following either long inspiration or expiration with the accompanying muscular tension. Sometimes, however, this relaxation was not total.

Modifications of cardiac activity were of various kinds. Acceleration of the cardiac rhythm up to 130 or 150 was very common, although sporadic extra systolic action was very uncommon. The pulse showed changes not only of rhythm but also of amplitude. The heart beat showed variations of intensity indicating both hypotonicity and hypertension of the heart action. There was observed to be displacement of the heart in relation to the mediastinal cavity. Such displacement generally coincided with moments of silence as observed by auscultation and a silent radial pulse but a feeble humoral pulse; the ECG records in such instances were normal but registered a low voltage. The most curious modifications, according to Brosse, were modifications in amplitude of various portions of the ECG. These changes might last for several seconds or several minutes. Some specific changes noted on various occasions were: an absence of the P part of the wave with the rest of the ECG record normal; a flattening of the T part of the wave so that it would have the appearance of a P wave; progressive suppression of the R part and accentuation of the S part of the wave.

The most extreme case of modified cardiac activity observed by Brosse involved generalized low ECG voltage recorded from the electrodes in the Lead I position. In this particular case, initially a very superficial respiration accompanied a normal ECG. A few seconds later there was an accentuation of all of the waves of the ECG and of the pulse image. Two minutes later a very low voltage was observed in all the waves of the ECG and towards the tenth minute of examination there followed a further considerable reduction of voltage and pulse and total cessation of respiratory activity. Finally, only a low voltage fibrillation effect was detected in the ECG. Subsequent to these very low amplitude fibrillation records in the ECG, whose duration was not stated, the record was normal.

Attempts by Yogi Ramananda (of Andhra) at stopping the heart were studied at the All-India Institute of Medical Science in New Delhi by Wenger.[28] The attempts involved retention of breath for about 15 seconds, after either inspiration or expiration, with closed glottis and strongly contracted chest and abdominal muscles. Radial pulse was feeble and heart sounds were inaudible; neck veins were distended. The ECG showed that heart contractions continued, but with certain modifications. There was a slight right axis deviation when the breath was retained after inspiration, and a corresponding left axis deviation when the breath was retained after expiration. During maintained inspiration the QRS potential was found to decrease in lead I and increase in lead III, while during maintained expiration the QRS potential was found to increase in lead I and decrease in lead III. X-ray examination revealed a decrease in the maximum transverse measurement of the heart, from a norm of 12 cm. to 11 cm. during the attempts following inspiration and to 11.5 cm. during the attempts following expiration. Plethysmographic recordings showed that finger pulse remained detectable during the heart stoppage attempts, and that finger pulse volume increased immediately after them. Blood pressure (brachial) also increased after the attempts, in one case from 130/96 mm. Hg. to 210/100 mm. Hg. These transient blood pressure increases were accompanied by transient increases in respiration rate, pulse rate and depth, and loudness of heart sounds. A few seconds after the attempts, heart rate returned to normal. Wenger's explanation of these attempts was that striated muscle activity altered cardiac function. It was suggested that the initial period, which involved strong abdominal contraction and breath arrest with closed glottis, precipitated an increase in intra-thoracic pressure which would accordingly limit the venous blood influx; hence, though the heart would contract there would be less blood for it to pump.

Wenger also studied N. R. Upadhyaya, a student of yoga for five years, in his attempts to slow the heart. The subject applied *uddiyana* and *jalanhara bandhas* (abdominal and chin locks) while in a supine position with a 4-5 inch thick rolled towel placed under the lumbar area of the spine and with the feet drawn toward the buttocks. In 6 trials the longest heart period noted was 2.9 seconds; the initial range of heart period had been .6 - .9 seconds and the heart period just after the maneuver was .8 seconds. Figure 2.27 shows the last 10 heart periods during this trial. The ECG record showed an increase in the P - R interval and, a few beats before termination of the maneuver, a decrease or disappearance of the P wave.

This same subject was studied at Kaivalyadhama by Bhole.[29] In 8 experiments he found that the subject's maximum heart period ranged from 2.9 seconds to 5.6 seconds. X-ray examination revealed a slight dilation of the heart. Bhole remarked that the hypothesis of increased intra-thoracic pressure in this case does not seem to be applicable, since in fact decreased intra-thoracic pressures have been measured in *uddiyana bandha* in other experiments. (See Figure 1.6.) An alternate hypothesis is that the subject increased vagal tone; it is known that an increase in the rate of stimulation by the vagus nerve of the heart's pacemaker center results in a decrease in the rate of heart contraction. Bhole accepted the vagal stimulation hypothesis as probable and termed the control to be semi-voluntary rather than completely voluntary.

We will now consider the observations by Elmer E. Green,[30] at the Menninger Foundation, of cardiac functioning with Swami Rama as the subject. In one experiment a sudden increase in heart rate was preceded by an ECG record notable in that it showed a T wave amplitude greater than the R wave amplitude. In another experiment the heart rate was slowed gradually from 75 beats per minute to 50 beats per minute with otherwise no particular change in the ECG. In a third experiment Swami Rama initiated a 17 second period of atrial flutter in which the ECG recorded a frequency of 300 beats per minute. A professor of cardiology said that this type of ECG record is "sometimes seen in patients and is associated with loss of blood flow in fainting or death." This atrial flutter was not initiated by a muscular action. Correlates of these heart rate experiments with Swami Rama were the low amplitude of the EEG and the decrease in respiratory activity. According to Swami Rama, an initial step in establishing control over internal bodily activities is to establish a pattern of even breathing in which a rate of only one or two breaths per minute can be maintained without discomfort.

A 12-lead ECG record was monitored by L. K. Kothari and colleagues[31] during a prolonged (7 days) confinement demonstration by a yogi at the Tagore Medical College and Hospital in Udaipur, India. One hour before closing the pit in which the yogi was confined there was in the yogi's ECG "normal sinus rhythm; heart rate was 106 per minute, PR interval was .16 second, QRS interval was .08 second, and there was an upright T wave." After the yogi had been confined for 29 hours, there was "severe sinus tachycardia with a heart rate of 250 per minute, a PR interval of .12 second, a QRS of .06 second, and a high uptake of the ST segment." After 30 hours the ECG record showed, in all leads, "a straight line with no electrical disturbance. This is continued for the next 5 days." On the eighth day, ½ hour before the pit was opened, the ECG record appeared: "sinus tachycardia is in evidence with a heart rate of 142 per minute, slightly prolonged PR interval of .20 second, a QRS interval of .06 second, and an upright T wave." Two hours after coming out of the pit, the yogi showed an ECG record whose wave characteristics were the same as those noted prior to confinement. (All ECG wave characteristics detailed above are from Lead II.) It would be of interest to replicate this experiment with consideration being given to such factors as skin resistance changes, which may affect ECG records. The subject's body temperature (oral) at termination was 94.6° F, and the subject experienced severe shivering for 2 hours.

For a fuller understanding of such studies as the two described above, a revision of physiological conceptualizations may be required, resulting from collaboration between physiologists and those students of yoga adept at control of internal process.

E. Blood Pressure

The pressure, or force per unit area, with which blood is propelled through the blood vessels is called the blood pressure. In the discussion of blood flow alterations, we noted various evidence supporting the view that during the performance of an asana variations in regional blood flow occur. (See Figures 2.3, 2.4, 2.5.) Similarly, in the performance of various yoga practices regional variations in blood pressure may be expected. Some data are available on such variations.

In studies by Rao, [32] both post-tibial and brachial blood pressures were noted as subjects sequentially assumed horizontal supine, erect standing, headstand, and horizontal supine positions. Systolic brachial blood pressure was less during an erect standing position than during a horizontal supine position, and was greater during *shirshasana* (headstand) than during a horizontal supine position. During the headstand, there was a decrease in post-tibial systolic pressure, in contrast to the increase in brachial systolic pressure. Diastolic and mean blood pressure readings generally followed the systolic blood pressure in direction and magnitude of change. The magnitude of changes in post-tibial pressure were considerably greater than the magnitude of changes in brachial pressure. In fact, the pressure measured at the ankle dropped almost to zero during the headstand posture. (See Figures 2.28 and 2.29.)

Swami Kuvalayananda[33] measured brachial blood pressure before, during and after 11 subjects practiced *shirshasana* (headstand), *sarvangasana* (shoulder stand) and *matsyasana* (fish posture). (See Figures 2.30, 2.31, and 2.32; the graphs are from mean values computed from the individual scores reported.) The general trend was for readings to be higher during practice of the asana than during sittings before and after the posture. The magnitude of the increase was greatest in *sarvangasana* and definitely less in both *shirshasana* and *matsyasana*. The increase during *shirshasana* is very close to that increase noted by Rao. Although increases in brachial blood pressure are perhaps expected during the headstand and shoulder stand, which are inverted postures, the increase noted during the fish posture, in which the body is not inverted, deserves further investigation.

After serious yoga students practiced *shavasana* (corpse posture) relaxation for a few minutes, their brachial blood pressure was almost the same as before *shavasana*.[34] (See Figure 2.33.) The subjects in this instance were normotensive. The same subjects showed small changes in blood pressure during certain breathing practices as compared to during a pre-practice period. Mean systolic pressure increased by 6 mm. Hg. during *bhastrika* (bellows) and 12 mm. Hg. during *kapalabhati* (skull-shining), and decreased slightly during *ujjayi*. Hyperventilation increased systolic pressure by about 4 mm. Hg. These changes are less than changes noted above in *shirshasana* (headstand), *sarvangasana* (shoulder stand) and *matsyasana* (fish posture).

Confinement experiments with various individuals, whether experienced or not in yoga practices, have found that blood pressure is essentially unchanged until the ambient concentration of carbon dioxide reaches about 5% at which time there is rapid increase in blood pressure.[35]

The effect of a program involving yoga practices on resting blood pressure has been considered by several investigators. The interest has usually been in subjects with high blood pressure, but before considering such studies we will briefly note studies involving normotensive subjects.

Gopal[36] noted the blood pressure before and after the performance of standard physical exercises (20 jumps and 20 sit-ups) by a group trained in hatha yoga for six months and a group that regularly engaged in light exercise. Both groups showed higher mean systolic pressure after the standard exercises than before, a greater increase being seen in the yoga group. Mean diastolic pressure decreased slightly for the yoga group and remained unchanged for the other group. None of the differences was reported to be statistically significant. (See Figure 2.36.)

The 12 normal subjects studied by Udupa [37] decreased average systolic blood pressure after 3 months of hatha yoga practices but returned to the pre-experiment value after 6 months. The average changes involved were small. (See Figure 2.37.)

Another subject studied by Udupa[38] showed a decrease in systolic blood pressure (measured with subject in sitting position) of 20 mm. Hg. after 3 months of daily practice of *sarvangasana* (shoulder stand), *matsyasana* (fish posture) and *halasana* (plow posture); lesser decreases (11 mm. Hg.) were noted when systolic and diastolic blood pressures were measured with the subject in standing position. Blood pressure changes in 2 subjects after 3 months practice of *suryanamaskar* (sun salutation) and in one subject after 3 months practice of *shirshasana* (headstand) and *mayurasana* (peacock posture) were generally of small magnitude and were variable in direction. (See Figures 2.38 and 2.39.)

In contrast to the small changes in resting blood pressure observed in normotensive subjects who practiced yoga, there are observations of significant decreases in resting blood pressure of hypertensives who practiced *shavasana* (corpse posture). Because of the predominance of hypertension as an ailment, the serious circulatory ailments statistically correlated with hypertensive segments of the population, and the lack of understanding of essential hypertension, it is an encouraging result of research in yoga that considerable evidence has been found suggesting that a program of relaxation and/or meditation may be helpful in lowering blood pressure in hypertensive patients and in maintaining blood pressure control while decreasing the level of drug therapy. This evidence has been reported by Dr. K. K. Datey and by Dr. Chandra H. Patel involving subjects who primarily practiced a form of *shavasana* relaxation and by Dr. Herbert Benson in studies involving subjects who practiced meditation. The effect of meditational programs on blood pressure in hypertensives will be considered in the second half of this book. (See Section C of Chapter 5.)

Datey's study[39] at the King Edward Memorial Hospital in Bombay involved a group of 47 hypertensive patients (32 essential hypertensives, 12 renal, 3 arteriosclerotic) whose average age was 46 years. There were 37 men and 10 women. The original (i.e., before any kind of treatment, drug or otherwise) blood pressure averaged 186 mm. Hg. for systolic, 115 mm. Hg. for diastolic. The patients were divided for the purpose of data evaluation into 3 categories according to their history of antihypertensive drug therapy. One group (10 subjects) had not received any such drug therapy. Twenty-two patients whose blood pressure was well-controlled by drugs comprised the second group and 15 subjects whose blood pressure was inadequately controlled in spite of drugs comprised the third group. The drug requirements of those in the second and third groups had been stabilized over a two-year period in the hospital's Hypertension Clinic. The details of *shavasana* as employed by Datey in training hypertensive patients were described as follows. The subject assumed the supine position of *shavasana* (corpse posture).

> The eyes were closed with eyelids drooping. Patient is taught slow, rhythmic, diaphragmatic breathing with a short pause after each inspiration and a long pause after each expiration. After establishing the rhythm he is asked to attend to his sensation at the nostrils, the coolness of the inspired air and the warmth of the expired air. This procedure helps to keep the patient inwardly alert and to forget his usual thoughts, thus becoming less conscious of the external environment, thereby attaining relaxation. The patient is asked to relax muscles so he is able to feel the heaviness of different parts of his body. This is achieved automatically once the patient learns the exercise.

The practice involves conscious relaxation of various muscle groups, in analogy to the general procedures in practicing an asana whereby one focuses his attention on and consciously relaxes those regions of tension emphasized by the particular asana; in *shavasana*, as there is minimal tension due to positional factors, the objective is reduction of ambient muscular tension. Rhythmic breathing, it may be recalled, is viewed as an important tool in gaining control over internal functions.

Most patients adequately learned *shavasana* relaxation in about 3 weeks of practice. In the data presented (see Figure 2.40), however, the duration of the before-after interval is not stated. Antihypertensive drug dosages were decreased where this was deemed consistent with blood pressure control by the attending physicians.

The first group (no drug therapy) showed a statistically significant (p < .05) change in mean blood pressure from 134 to 107 mm. Hg. (Mean blood pressure equals diastolic blood pressure plus one-third the pulse pressure.) Nine of the 10 subjects showed a decrease in mean blood pressure, the amount of the decrease ranging from 22 to 43 mm. Hg. One subject increased mean blood pressure by 9 mm. Hg. The second group, whose blood pressure had been controlled with drug therapy, neither was expected to nor did show significant change in mean blood pressure. The satisfactory blood pressure level was maintained, however, while drug requirements decreased in some cases. In fact, drug requirements decreased by an average of 68% and by at least 33% in 13 of the 22 patients in the second group (p<.05); only 3 of the other 9 patients were regular in their practice of *shavasana*. The third group showed an average decrease in mean blood pressure from 120 to 110 mm. Hg. Further, the drug requirement was decreased by 71% in 6 of these 15 patients; of the 5 remaining patients who practiced *shavasana* regularly and correctly, the drug requirement was unchanged in 3 cases and increased slightly in 2 cases. Four of those 9 patients with no clinically significant (greater than 33%) decrease in drug requirement did show decreases in mean blood pressure.

Of all those subjects with essential hypertension, 62% responded favorably to *shavasana* treatment; 42% of those with renal hypertension responded favorably; none of the 3 with arteriosclerotic hypertension showed improvement. The 20% difference between essential and renal hypertension groups was not statistically significant.

Patel reported in 3 studies the utility of a yoga relaxation program in the management of hypertension. The method of yoga relaxation (*shavasana*, corpse posture) employed was similar to that used by Datey. Subjects concentrated on attaining smoothly rhythmic breath, practiced voluntary relaxation of the musculature, and then remained alert by mental repetition of some word in cadence with inspiration and expiration. During yoga relaxation periods subjects were provided audio-feedback of finger skin resistence. (EMG feedback was used with some subjects.) In her first study Dr. Patel[40] chose 20 patients from a suburban London group general practice. All but one were on antihypertensive therapy. There were 11 women and 9 men; the average age was 57.35 years; the average duration of hypertension was 6.8 years. The etiology of hypertension was classified as essential in 14 patients, renal in 2, essential following pregnancy toxemia in 3 and intracranial in 1. The blood pressure readings before and after 3 months of thrice-weekly half-hour yoga and biofeedback sessions may be summarized as follows. (See Figure 2.41.) The average value of the mean blood pressure of 121 mm. Hg. before the treatment decreased to 101mm. Hg. after treatment; in 19 subjects mean blood pressure decreased. In addition to blood pressure decrease, the total drug requirement decreased by 41%. Five patients terminated their antihypertensive drug usage and 7 decreased their drug requirement by 33% to 60%. In 4 subjects whose drug requirement did not decrease, mean blood pressure decreased by 17 to 30 mm. Hg. Four patients significantly reduced neither drug requirement nor mean blood pressure; these were all classified as essential hypertensives.

Dr. Patel followed up this treatment group for 12 months.[41] Each month subjects came in for blood pressure checks. They were encouraged to continue practicing the yoga relaxation at home. Some patients who found this daily practice inconvenient substituted other procedures involving checking for tension and

relaxing in response to such environmental cues as ringing tele-
phones and red traffic lights. Concurrent with this 12 month
follow-up of the yoga-biofeedback group, Dr. Patel studied a
control group. This control group was matched to the treatment
group with respect to age and sex; average values for duration of
hypertension and original systolic and diastolic blood pressure
before drug treatment were also nearly the same in both groups.
All but 2 in the control group were on antihypertensive drug
therapy. Three months of thrice-weekly blood pressure checks for
this group were intended to control against drops in blood
pressure due to placebo effects. Where the treatment group had
been trained with yoga relaxation and biofeedback, the control
group was instructed to rest on a couch. The control group was
followed up for 9 months. Drug dosages were adjusted so blood
pressure remained in a satisfactory range.

Whereas for the treatment group the initial 3 months had
yielded significant decreases (p < .001) in systolic and diastolic
blood pressure, blood pressure changes in the control group were
not significant in the initial 3 month period. Blood pressures
at the end of the follow-up periods did not for either group differ
significantly from those after the initial 3 month periods. (See
Figure 2.42.) Drug requirements in the control group changed
little during the first 6 months. A decrease of drug dosage for one
patient in the first 3 months and an increase for one patient in
the second 3 months were noted during follow-up of the treatment group.

A subsequent, more formally designed, experiment by
Patel[42] confirmed that a yoga-biofeedback program can lower the
blood pressure of hypertensives. Thirty-four hypertensive patients
were assigned randomly to one of two groups, group A or group
B. Group A contained 6 men and 11 women; group B contained
7 men and 10 women. Average age for group A was 59.5 years,
for group B 58.6 years. Fifteen from group A and all from group
B were using antihypertensive drugs; one in group A was on

tranquilizers and one was untreated. Initial average blood pressure was about the same in both groups. Patients were requested not to change their drug therapy during the experiment.

The experiment had two 6-week phases separated by 5 months. In phase 1, group A proceeded with yoga-biofeedback training and group B proceeded with uninstructed relaxation (similar to the control group described above). In phase 2, group A received no further attention but group B was now instructed in the yoga-biofeedback procedure. The difference between group A and group B in before-after changes in blood pressure for each phase was significant. As expected, the group being treated with yoga relaxation and biofeedback showed considerable decrease in blood pressure while the other group showed little change. (See Figure 2.43.) Group A retained the lower blood pressure for the duration of the experiment.

F. Blood Composition

Through the uncounted ramifications of the circulatory vessels, the fluid tissue of the body is made accessible to each living cell. Material exchanges are made between blood and other tissues. Investigators have already made a few preliminary observations of various blood constituents in persons who have practiced hatha yoga, and these will be detailed below (with the exception of certain constituents more properly considered in Chapter 4).

When a sample of blood is centrifuged the so-called formed elements, mostly red blood cells and white blood cells, settle below a clear straw-colored fluid, the plasma. Red cells settle below white cells, and the percentage of the blood volume consisting of red blood cells is called the hematocrit. Typical hematocrit values are between 45% and 50%. Dhanaraj[43] reports that 6 weeks of daily hatha yoga practices gave statistically significant ($p < .05$) changes in average hematocrit reading in 17

subjects, from 45.9% before to 47.5% after. Six weeks of detraining did not further significantly change the hematocrit in
this yoga group. Values noted in the hematocrit for a group practicing the 5BX exercise program for 6 weeks and for a control
group did not change significantly. (See Figure 2.44.) The
statistical significances for changes in the red blood cell count
and in the hemoglobin content of the blood were similar, showing
increases in red blood cell count and hemoglobin after 6 weeks
of hatha yoga. The values for all groups were about the same
as or slightly higher than values considered to be average. (See
Figures 2.45 and 2.46.)

A report[44] has been made of blood tests administered to
asthmatic patients before and after a 4 or 6 week treatment
based on yoga practices. The treatment was administered by
M. V. Bhole, M.D., at the Gupta Yogic Hospital at Kaivalyadhama,
Lonavala, India. Altogether 104 patients were involved in the
study; they suffered from asthma and did not show heart, kidney
or liver complications. After a control period of either 2 or 4
weeks, patients undertook the yogic treatment, which included
asanas, relaxation, and certain breathing and internal cleansing
practices prescribed according to the characteristics and history
of the individual patient. Increases were reported in hemoglobin
content, red blood cell count and lymphocyte count, while there
were decreases in total leukocyte (white blood cell) count and in
the count of polymorphs, eosinophils, basophils, and monocytes
(various white blood cell types). The changes in hemoglobin
content, total white blood cell count, and lymphocyte count were
statistically significant ($p < .05$). Elsewhere[45] Dr. Bhole summarized the changes in the asthmatic patients. Seventy-six per
cent of the patients had no asthmatic attacks during the treatment
period and showed improvement as determined by laboratory and
clinical assessment. (This latter article presents details of the
treatment procedure and certain information gleaned from follow-
up interviews.)

The total leukocyte count was seen by Udupa[46] to decrease after 3 months of certain hatha yoga practices. Since only 4 subjects were involved, no statistical inferences were warranted. In studying this data (See Figure 2.47) one might consider that normal leukocyte counts usually range between 7,000 and 9,000 per cubic centimeter of blood, and that variations outside this range may occur in a given individual.

The blood plasma consists of 91% water and 9% solid matter. From the vast diversity of substances composing the solid matter of plasma, researchers have assayed protein, urea, creatinine, sugar and cholesterol contents in relation to hatha yoga practices. In particular, attention has been paid to plasma proteins, which include albumins, globulins and fibrinogen. An average value (in grams per 100 milliliters of plasma) for normal plasma protein is 7, of which albumins contribute 4.2, globulins 2.5 and fibrinogen .3. *Serum* is plasma with the fibrinogen, which is involved in clotting, removed.

The procedural details of the two studies by Udupa have been mentioned earlier in this chapter. Udupa's 1971 study involved 12 males, average age 23 years; his 1975 study involved 4 males, average age 20 years. The biochemical studies done by Gopal[47] involved subjects whose mean age was 31.5 years. Gopal's subjects practiced *asanas, pranayamas, mudras* (seals), *bandhas* (locks) and *kriyas* (cleansing practices). Training in asanas included *padmasana* (lotus posture), *siddhasana* (accomplished posture), *bhujangasana* (cobra posture), *shalabhasana* (locust posture), *ardha-shalabhasana* (half-locust posture), *dhanurasana* (bow posture), *halasana* (plow posture), *paschimottanasana* (posterior stretching posture), *ardha-matsyendrasana* (half-spinal twist), *mayurasana* (peacock posture), and *shavasana* (corpse posture). Training in other yoga practices included *viparitakarani* (inverted action), *sarvangasana* (shoulder stand), *matsyasana* (fish posture), *shirshasana* (headstand), *yoga mudra* (symbol of yoga), *uddiyana-bandha* (abdominal lock), *jalandhara bandha* (chin lock), *mula*

bandha (anal lock), *nauli, nadi shodhana* (alternate nostril breathing), *ujjayi, bhastrika* (bellows) and *kapalabhati* (skull-shining).
Subjects were tested for various components of blood chemistry initially and after 1, 3 and 6 months of yoga practice. For each component of blood chemistry, Gopal reported the number of males and females who showed no change, or an increase or a decrease, and the average and range of the increases and decreases.
The 1-month changes for 5 males and 7 females were presented, and three- and six-month changes for 8 males and 14 females.

Total serum protein (Udupa, 1971) was seen to have decreased somewhat from its initial value at the end of 3 months of hatha yoga, but then to have increased significantly ($p < .05$) at the end of 6 months of yoga. (See Figure 2.48.) Serum globulin showed a decrease after 3 months and a larger increase after 6 months, while serum albumin increased after 3 months then decreased a lesser amount after 6 months. (See Figures 2.49 and 2.50.) Serum globulin and albumin changes were not statistically significant ($p < .05$). Average values for total serum protein and for serum globulin were lower than the values mentioned above as normal, while serum albumin was close to normal.

Gopal found no change in serum protein in over 50% of the subjects after 1, 3 or 6 months of hatha yoga; where change was noted, it was predominately an increase, in the range of .5 to 1.8 gm./100 ml. (see Figure 2.51). In plasma albumin, more subjects increased than did not change, and still fewer decreased (see Figure 2.52). In plasma globulins 50% of the subjects had shown a decrease after one month of yoga although more people showed a decrease than showed an increase after 3 and 6 months; 59% showed no change in plasma globulins after these intervals. (See Figure 2.53.)

None of Gopal's subjects showed any change in the level of creatinine and urea in the blood after 1, 3 or 6 months of yoga practice. Creatinine and urea are two sources of the non-protein nitrogen found in blood plasma. (See Figure 2.54.)

Blood sugar, primarily glucose dissolved in the plasma, is made available to body cells which oxidize it to provide energy stores for their functioning. When several hours have elapsed after food ingestion, the blood sugar level (fasting blood sugar) will normally be about 60-80 mg./100 ml.

Udupa (1971) found a statistically significant (p < .05) decrease of about 10.5 mg./100 ml. in the fasting blood sugar of subjects after three months of hatha yoga; after 6 months a slightly greater decrease was seen. (See Figure 2.55.) The final average of 63 mg./100 ml. is at the low end of the normal range as defined above. In the 4 subjects studied by Udupa (1975), no consistent change in blood sugar was seen after 3 months of selected yogic or non-yogic practices. (See Figure 2.56.) It may be noted that all values are considerably higher than the normal fasting blood sugar levels mentioned above. Gopal reported that after 6 months of hatha yoga, the blood sugar level had decreased for half the subjects he studied and had not changed for the other half. (See Figure 2.57.) No more than 20% of the subjects showed an increase in blood sugar after 1 month or 6 months. Decreases ranged between 11 and 59 mg./100 ml., but the actual levels were unreported.

Cholesterol, a compound associated with but chemically different from fats, is found in all body tissues. Relations between the serum cholesterol level and various common circulatory diseases have been studied by medical researchers. Upper bounds for normal serum cholesterol have been suggested to be 180 or 200 mg./100 ml.

Twelve subjects of Udupa (1971) averaged a statistically significant decrease (p < .01) in serum cholesterol after three months of hatha yoga. After 6 months the serum cholestrol had increased, but not back to its initial level. All average values reported were normal. (See Figure 2.58.) Three of 4 other subjects studied by Udupa (1975) showed a decrease in plasma cholesterol after 3 months of selected yogic and non-yogic

practices.   (See Figure 2.59.)   The subject whose cholesterol
increased was practicing *suryanamaskar* (sun salutation), although
in another subject practicing *suryanamaskar* the blood cholesterol
decreased.   One subject's plasma cholesterol decreased from the
value of 196.9 mg %, which is high according to one suggestion,
to the value of 104.5 mg.%, which is considered in the normal
range;   this subject practiced *sarvangasana* (shoulder stand),
matsyasana (fish posture) and *halasana* (plow posture).   After 6
months of hatha yoga, blood cholesterol had decreased for 55%,
not changed for 40% and increased for 5% of the subjects studied
by Gopal.   (See Figure 2.60.)   The range of decreases after 6
months was 10-72 mg.%, with more females (9 of 14) showing
decrease than males (3 of 8).

·3·

Respiratory Responses to Hatha Yoga

Respiratory variables have been among the most frequently measured physiological variables in scientific studies of yoga, partially as a result of the concern in yoga practices, especially in the pranayama practices, with the breathing system. It should be remembered, however, that what pranayama practices have been designed to control is not breathing patterns but pranic, or energy, patterns. Control of the breath reportedly can, with expert guidance, lead to control of prana. This distinction between prana and breath results in certain concerns of pranayama that have not reached the general attention of respiratory physiologists. One such conern is that of nostril dominance, which has been verified and investigated in a preliminary manner by physiologists: this work will be the first topic of concern to us in this chapter. The remainder of the chapter will review effects of yoga on conventional respiratory variables. These will be divided into the large categories of respiratory patterns, air movement, and gas transfer.

A. Nostril Dominance

A model of the respiratory system is that of two elastic bags, the lungs, in the chest cavity with passageways to the exterior of the body. On its way to the lungs air normally enters through the 2 nostrils, then traverses the nasal passages, the pharyngeal tube and the trachea, which bifurcates into the 2 bronchi, which enter the lungs. This pathway is followed in the opposite order by air from the lungs leaving the body.

Air which enters or leaves the nostrils consists of 2 parts, that which moves through the left naris and that which moves through the right naris. For a given individual at a given time, the relative amount of air moving through each nostril may be the same, or it may be greater through one nostril than through the other. Yoga asserts certain psychological and behavioral tendencies to be correlated with these 3 states, (that is, right nostril dominant, left nostril dominant, and equality of nostril activity). There are further assertions in yoga texts concerning natural rhythmic changes from the dominance of one nostril to that of the other; such changes are said to occur every 2 or 3 hours. It is said that the equal flow of breath through the 2 nostrils is the preferable condition for practicing meditation.

With a little practice a person can learn to discriminate in himself which nostril is active. Pratap[1] had 99 people do this and record the result for 2 months; the subjects noted the condition of nostril activity each day at 3-hour intervals, from 6 a.m. to 9 p.m. Most subjects were hospital patients. Statistical analysis of the data confirmed the variable nostril dominance, but could not be used to confirm the rhythmicity of change. Biotelemetry might be useful in gaining more information on this point.

In a series of observations by Bhole[2] on 75 men and 21 women, all in good health, the resting state nostril breathing pattern was determined. Here a tube from each nostril was attached to a device to record the force of breathing. In 47.8%

of the cases, breathing force was greater for the right nostril than for the left, while in 37.7% of the cases breathing force was greater for the left nostril. In only 14.5% of the cases was the breathing force of equal magnitude in the right and left nostril. (See Figure 3.1.)

If a particular mode of nostril dominance is preferable for a certain activity, then techniques to control nostril dominance would be of use. Two studies have investigated the efficacy of traditional yoga techniques developed for this purpose. The study by Bhole, mentioned above, considered the technique of *yoga danda*. Subjects were asked to place a crutch-like instrument (the *yoga danda*) under an armpit and to lean over and press it between the chest and the arm; this position was maintained for ten or fifteen minutes while breathing force from each nostril was recorded. The results suggest that the breathing force is increased in the nostril on the side opposite to the *yoga danda* and decreased in the nostril on the same side. (See Figure 3.2.) Rao[3] came to similar conclusions in studying *yoga danda*. Five healthy male subjects were involved. Measurements of ventilation per minute in each nostril were made after a subject had been in a position for 10 minutes. (See Figure 3.3.) The average values of right and left minute ventilation were the same after 10 minutes of sitting. After 10 minutes of sitting with a crutch under one arm, minute ventilation was greater through the nostril on the other side; the differences in right and left ventilation were statistically significant ($p < .03$).

Rao also studied the relative nostril minute ventilation in 3 horizontal postures. In supine posture, average minute ventilation was about the same through each nostril. "For the lateral postures, the subjects lay comfortably on a bed, the weight of the body being borne on the lateral aspect of the thigh, temporal region, shoulder, and arm." After 10 minutes in the right lateral position, the average minute ventilation was greater through the left nostril, and *vice versa* (i. e., the "up" nostril was more active); the differences were statistically significant (p<.05). (See Figure 3.4.)   Rao also found a positive correlation (r=.8) between nasal ventilation observed in subjects in lateral posture and that of subjects applying the *yoga danda*.   He asserts that variations in blood flow through the nasal mucosa account for variations in resistance to flow of air through the 2 nares.   He believes the mechanism involved in controlling these variations is the same for the 2 techniques he studied. The nature of this mechanism is not yet clear.

B. Respiratory Pattern

The rate at which breaths are taken has been measured in connection with a variety of yoga practices.   Other variables in addition to breath rate that will be considered in this section are breath-holding time, respiratory amplitude, and chest expansion measurements.

B.1 Breath Rate

Normal breath rate while resting is sometimes stated to be 16 breaths per minute.   The rate may be lower in supine rest, and this is sometimes called basal state for respiratory rate. A number of studies have found the basal breath rate to be lower in subjects who have practiced a routine of hatha yoga for some time.

Udupa[4] found that 6 months of a hatha yoga program resulted in statistically significant (p < .05) changes in basal breath rate.   Initially, the average for 12 subjects was 16.8 breaths per minute.   After 3 months, the mean respiration rate was 16.6, an insignificant change from the initial value (see Figure 3.5), but after 6 months the average was 13.4.   In another study by Udupa,[5] breath rate (standing at rest) increased in one subject and didn't change in another who practiced *suryanamaskar* (sun salutation) daily for 3 months. Breath rate (standing at rest) decreased from 24 to 19 in a subject who practiced *shirshasana* (headstand) and *mayurasana* (peacock posture) for 3 months. Little change in breath rate was seen in a subject who practiced *sarvangasana* (shoulder stand), *matsyasana* (fish posture) and *halasana* (plow posture) for 3 months. (See Figure 3.6.)

A small, but statistically significant ($p < .05$), change was seen by Dhanaraj[6] in 17 subjects who practiced several asanas and a breathing exercise for 6 weeks. The decrease seen was from 11.3 to 10.1 breaths per minute in basal state. Another group who practiced the 5BX Program for Physical Fitness for a similar period showed a similar decrease in breath rate, while a control group showed no change. (See Figure 3.7.)

Gopal[7] found a great difference in basal breath rate between a group that had been trained in hatha yoga for 6 months and a group that was untrained in yoga but regularly engaged in long walks and light exercise games. The average basal breath rate for the yoga group was 10 breaths per minute, while that for the untrained group was 23. (See Figure 3.8.) Unfortunately, initial differences in breath rate between the groups were not stated. When breath rate was determined for these 2 groups before and after a standard physical exercise (20 jumps and 20 sit-ups), the increase in breath rate for the group trained in yoga was less than for the light exercise group untrained in yoga. (See Figure 3.9.)

Breath rate was also noted[8] during the practice of several asanas by these 2 groups. (See Figure 3.10) The lowest rate for both groups was seen during *shavasana* (corpse posture) and this was slightly below the basal rate noted above. The next lowest breath rate for both groups was seen in *dharmic asana* (symbol of yoga). For the trained group the highest (18) and next highest (16) breath rates were recorded in *ardha-matsyendrasana* (half-spinal twist) and *viparitakarani* (inverted action); these same 2 asanas gave, respectively, the next highest (30) and highest (32) breath rate averages for the untrained groups. The difference in breath rate between the 2 groups remained about the same (15) during practice of the sequence of asanas.

Measurements by Wenger,[9] Datey,[10] and Dhanaraj[11] reported that breath rate decreased during and after the practice of *shavasana* (corpse posture). In all these cases breath rate decreased to less than 10 breaths per minute. (See Figures 3.11 and 3.12.) We may recall that Datey was studying hypertensive patients.

Rao[12] found variations in breath rate in relation to body position. Five minutes in the erect standing position yielded a breath rate higher than in the horizontal supine position. Five minutes in *shirshasana* (headstand) did not change breath rate from its value in the erect standing position: it still was higher, by a statistically significant difference ($p < .05$), than the prior value in the horizontal supine position. (See Figure 3.13.)

Data presented in the last few paragraphs support the idea that breath rate increases during the practice of asanas (except *shavasana* [corpse posture], though to a lesser degree than in standard physical exercise. Pranayama practices often involve attention to the rate of breathing. In most yogic breathing practices, including those involved in relaxation, one objective is to decrease the breath rate. Of course, a person can temporarily decrease his breath rate by simply holding his breath, but this would normally be followed by the other extreme of rapid breathing. In yogic breathing exercises, breath rate decreases occur only gradually, over a period of several months of daily practice. After such training, periods of slow breathing do not require subsequent respiratory compensation.

Both Miles[13] and Rao[14] noted several respiratory variables before, during and after *ujjayi*. *Ujjayi* involves a deep inspiration, a retention of breath and then a deep expiration. In the subject studied by Miles, the breath was held after inspiration for about 40 seconds; after expiration there began without pause the inspiration of the next round of *ujjayi*. As might be expected, *ujjayi* would involve a very small number of breaths per minute. In data from this subject, the mean for 5 twenty-minute trials was 1.26 breaths per minute. In the minutes prior to the *ujjayi* practice, breaths per minute averaged about 22; in the minutes subsequent to the *ujjayi* practice, there were approximately 19 breaths per minute in the first minute after *ujjayi* and then 20 or 21 in the next several minutes. (See Figure 3.14.) The breath rate in basal state for this subject was about 16 per minute. In the subject studied by Rao, breath rate during 10 minutes of *ujjayi* was 1.5 at a low altitude (520 meters) and 3.0 at a high altitude (3800 meters). During normal breathing, the breath rate was higher at the low altitude. (See Figure 3.15.)

Miles also studied *kapalabhati* (skull-shining) and *bhastrika* (bellows) as practiced by his subject. *Kapalabhati* consists of rapid abdominal diaphragmatic breathing in which there is no retention. Instructions in the exercise sometimes say that about 2 breaths per second or 120 breaths per minute should be maintained for a minute or so. Over a twenty-five-minute period in which this rapid breathing was alternated with periods of spontaneous breathing, the breath rate averaged 80 or more per minute in the first period and 12½ per minute in the second. The mean number of breaths was lower in the minutes before *kapalabhati* began, about 15 breaths per minute, than afterwards, when it was about 19 per minute. The variety of *bhastrika* (bellows) breathing studied by Miles consists of alternation of *kapalabhati* (skull-shining) breathing with *ujjayi* breathing. In the subject studied by Miles the period of *bhastrika* began with *ujjayi*—the inhalation, retention and exhalation—and continued with an inhalation followed by about 20 cycles of the *kapalabhati*-type breathing followed by a deep exhalation and subsequent *ujjayi* cycle. In a 25-minute period of *bhastrika*, in the *kapalabhati* part of the exercise it was noted there was a mean number of breaths of 21 per 10 seconds while in the *ujjayi* part the mean number of breaths was 1.3 per minute. Breath rate was slightly higher in the minute preceding the *bhastrika* period (21.2) than in the minute following the *bhastrika* period (18.7).

Breath rate has been monitored in subjects during confinement experiments. Anand[15] found that the breath rate for a trained subject was stable at about 20/minute for 8 hours of confinement; during the last 2 hours of confinement, when carbon dioxide content in the confinement box was over 4.4% and oxygen content was under 15.8%, the subject's breath rate increased to 26/minute. This contrasted to a gradual steady increase over the period of containment for 2 normal subjects. In the Kaivalyadhama confinement studies, breath rate was found by Karambelkar[16] to change only slightly until the ambient carbon dioxide concentration was 5% the breath rate increased when the carbon dioxide content of inspired air was greater than 5%.

Rao[17] reported that the normal respiration rate of Yogi Ramananda of Mysore in the beginning of confinement experiments was about 16 per minute. Later during the confinement, the spirogram showed irregular respirations at about 1 per minute. Ballentine and Gibbons[18] reported a respiratory rate of 9 per minute in Yogi Ramananda during the first 7 minutes of an oxygen tent confinement study. From 15.0 minutes to 33.0 minutes (the end) of confinement, respiratory rate was 1.2 per minute. The percentages of oxygen and carbon dioxide present at the 15th minute were 16.35 and 4.42 respectively, and at the 33rd minute were 12.8 and 7.14. The absence of hyperventilation by the subject in an atmosphere unusually high in carbon dioxide suggests an unusual control by the subject over his respiratory rate.

B.2 Breath Holding Time

Now, we consider the variable of breath holding time. In a study[19] over several years of the effect of a three-week program of hatha yoga on physical education students, there was seen to be a statistically significant increase of 15 seconds in breath holding time (p<.01). The range of increase was seen to be from 10 to 22 seconds.

Gopal[20] found that a group of subjects trained in yoga for 6 months or more had a slightly lower duration of breath holding time than a group of subjects who had frequent exercise in long walks and light games, though the average difference of 3.3 seconds was not statistically significant. The untrained group had a mean breath holding time of 57.7 seconds and the trained group a mean breath holding time of 54.4 seconds. (See Figure 3.16.) Dhanaraj[21] reported that 6 weeks' practice of 15 minutes of hatha yoga daily produced a statistically significant (p < .05) change in breath holding time. (See Figure 3.17.) This increase of 12 seconds from 54 seconds to 66 seconds was lost, however, when yoga practice was discontinued: after 6 weeks of de-training, the average breath holding time was 57 seconds. Another group that practiced the 5BX Program for Physical Fitness for 6 weeks showed a much smaller, yet statistically significant, 4 second increase in breath holding time.

Udupa[27] found similar evidence for increase in breath holding time as a result of a practice of yoga postures and breathing exercises. After 3 months of such a routine the initial mean breath holding time of 74.8 seconds for 12 subjects increased to 99.3 seconds (p < .01); after 6 months a further slight increase was seen. (See Figure 3.18.) Two subjects, studied by Udupa, who practiced *suryanamaskar* (sun salutation) for three months showed increases in breath holding time of 11 and 6 seconds. (See Figure 3.19.) No changes in breath holding time were noted in a subject practicing *shirshasana* (headstand) and *mayurasana* (peacock posture) for 3 months or in a subject practicing *sarvangasana* (shoulder stand), *matsyasana* (fish posture) and *halasana* (plow posture) for 3 months.

Moses[23] measured breath holding time before and after a ten-week hatha yoga class for one group and 10 weeks of physical education classes for a control group. When the 2 groups were compared, the yoga group increased, by an amount significantly greater than the increase for the control group, the breath holding time after full exhalation, after full inhalation preceded by hyperventilation, and after normal inhalation ($p < .05$). There was no significant difference between the groups in the increase of the breath holding time after full inhalation. (See Figure 3.20.)

B.3 Respiratory Amplitude

Pneumographic measurements were made by Gopal[24] on two groups, one trained in yoga and the other untrained in yoga. In normal rhythmic breathing, the thoracic amplitude of respiration was seen to be significantly different ($p < .05$) for the two groups; respiratory amplitude was greater in the group that had practiced hatha yoga for 6 months or more. (See Figure 3.21.) This same relation between average respiratory amplitude measurements of the 2 groups was maintained during the practice of various asanas.[25] In general, the pattern of respiratory amplitude change was similar as each group went through the sequence of asanas. (See Figure 3.22.) The greatest respiratory amplitude occurred during *dharmic asana* (symbol of yoga) for the trained group and during *ardha-matsyendrasana* (half-spinal twist) for the untrained group. Minimal amplitude of respiration occurred during *shavasana* (corpse posture) for the untrained group and during *sarvangasana* (shoulder stand) for the trained group.

During the practice of *shavasana* (corpse posture) a pneumographic record of one of Datey's hypertensive patients showed not only an increased amplitude with the decreased breath rate, but also a greater smoothness.[26] If we imagine the respiratory cycles as a roughly sinusoidal curve, then ordinarily there will be a jaggedness overlaying this sinusoidal shape, caused by numerous little jerks in the breath. An explicit instruction in yogic breathing practice is to see that there are no jerks in the breath, so that the breath may flow smoothly. A smoothly flowing breath is said by teachers of yoga to correlate with smoothness in the flow of thoughts. It would seem of interest to make more careful investigations of respiratory records, using techniques of power spectrum analysis that have proved useful in EEG studies, of this aspect of the respiratory pattern.

Even after a normal inspiration the chest may be further expanded. The magnitude of this chest expansion may be indicative of lung capacity. After 3 months of hatha yoga practice, the average value of chest expansion in 12 subjects studied by Udupa[27] was .9 cm. greater than before the practice; 3 more months increased mean chest expansion by .4 cm. more. The overall six-month change of 1.3 cm. was statistically significant (p < .05). (See Figure 3.23.) In the study by Dhanaraj[28] the mean chest expansion for 17 subjects after 6 weeks of hatha yoga was 1.8 cm. greater than the initial mean value. For a group practicing the 5BX Plan an increase of 1 cm. was seen. The changes for both groups were statistically significant (p < .01). (See Figure 3.24.)

Gopal[29] studied the effect of the *bandhas* (locks) on chest measurement changes. (See Figure 3.25.) Measurements were made on 52 subjects of various body types. The average increase in chest measurement over normal, after full inspiration, was seen to be greater when *bandhas* were applied than otherwise. Conversely, the average decrease in chest size over normal after full expiration was seen to be less when *bandhas* were applied than otherwise. The differences in chest measurement changes with and without application of the *bandhas* was found to be statistically significant (p < .01) in both cases (viz., inspiration and expiration). An interpretation of these latter results is that the *bandhas* (locks) serve as safety measures to reduce effects on various organ systems in the thoracic cavity.

C. Air Movement

The result of the rhythmic diaphragmatic, thoracic and abdominal movements in respiration is movement of air into and out of the lungs. Measurements of several aspects of this air movement have been made in connection with hatha yoga practices, and these will now be surveyed.

C.1 Tidal Volume

The amount of air inspired with a normal breath is called the tidal volume. An average value for tidal volume in the basal state is 500 ml. Tidal volume normally increases during activity. In subjects practicing *shirshasana* (headstand), Rao[30] found a statistically significant increase ($p < .05$) in tidal volume over that when subjects were in the horizontal supine position. (See Figure 3.26.) The headstand tidal volume was also greater than the erect standing tidal volume. Rao conjectured that this increased tidal volume, which resulted in an increased minute ventilation, (see Figure 3.31) was due to muscular effort required to maintain the headstand posture. If this conjecture is true, then it might be the case that increases in tidal volume would be less when *shirshasana* is practiced by an expert in hatha yoga.

In another study, Rao[31] found a rather high value, about 2 liters, for the tidal volume of a subject practicing *ujjayi*. (See Figure 3.27.) The value was slightly lower when *ujjayi* was practiced at a high altitude.

Dhanaraj[32] reports that tidal volume for subjects after practice of *shavasana* (corpse posture) was less than before the practice. (See Figure 3.28.) In contrast, tidal volume was greater after than before an equal period of supine rest by subjects untrained in yoga. The differences in both cases were statistically significant ($p < .05$.)

Two studies suggest that a program of hatha yoga may

increase basal state tidal volume. In both studies the yoga program included pranayama exercises. Basal tidal volume was
significantly different (p < .001) when Gopal [33] compared 2
groups, (see Figure 3.29) one which had been trained in
hatha yoga for a period of 6 months and another which had
not been so trained. (Pre-training values were not presented.)
In Dhanaraj's study,[34] (see Figure 3.30) basal tidal volume
changed significantly (p < .002) in the direction of increased tidal
volume after 6 weeks of hatha yoga practices. In a control group
and in a group practicing the 5BX exercises, there were no significant differences between the average values for tidal volume
before and after 6 weeks.

C.2 Minute Ventilation

Minute ventilation, or ventilation volume, is defined to be
the product of breath rate and tidal volume (assuming tidal
volume and breath volume to be constant over the interval of time
considered). Normally, it is about 8 liters per minute. Since there
was a slight increase in breath rate and a significant increase in
tidal volume during *shirshasana* (headstand) as observed by Rao,[35]
it follows that there would have been an increase in minute
ventilation during headstand. There was indeed a statistically
significant difference in average minute ventilation between the
headstand posture and the horizontal supine posture (p < .05).
(See Figure 3.31.)

Other studies of hatha yoga that present explicit values for
minute ventilation are those involving pranayama: Miles[36] noted
the ventilation in each of the 6 minutes before *ujjayi*, during the
ujjayi period and in each of the 6 minutes after *ujjayi*. (See
Figure 3.32.) In measurements with his subject on 5 days, there
was seen to be an increase in ventilation from about 9 liters
in the sixth minute before the *ujjayi* period to 14 liters in the last
minute before the *ujjayi* period. During the *ujjayi* period the

minute ventilation was fairly constant at 3.5 liters/minute. In the minutes following *ujjayi*, ventilation was fairly stable at between 8 and 9 liters/minute. Miles viewed the increase in ventilation prior to the *ujjayi* practice as a respiratory preparation for the practice. To know whether this respiratory preparation for *ujjayi* was a general phenomenon or a peculiarity of the subject studied by Miles would require the collection of more data. A subject studied by Rao[37] did, like Mile's subject, show a decrease of ventilation during *ujjayi*. (See Figures 3.33 and 3.34.) The decrease was from about 6 to 3 liters/minute at a low altitude (500 meters) and from 7.8 to 5.5 at a high altitude (3800 meters).

Miles reports the following figures on minute ventilation in his subject's practice of *kapalabhati* (skull-shining) and *bhastrika* (bellows). In *kapalabhati*, in the slow phase of spontaneous breathing, the ventilation varied between 1.8 and 5.9 liters per minute. In the fast part, ventilation averaged 18.3 liters per minute. In the 6 minutes before the *kapalabhati* period, the ventilation was rather low, ranging from 5 to 6.7, with an average of 6.2 liters/minute. Following *kapalabhati*, the ventilation was about the normal value of 8 liters/minute. In the six-minute period before the *bhastrika* exercise, the ventilation gradually increased from 7.8 liters in the 6th minute before the exercise to 10.9 liters in the minute before the exercise. For the *kapalabhati* part of the exercise, there was an average ventilation of 5.1 liters per 10 seconds; ventilation averaged 3.8 liters/minute in the *ujjayi* part. The ventilation volume ranged between 7.5 and 8.2 liters in each of the 6 minutes subsequent to *bhastrika*.

The normal movement of air, whether in basal state after a regimen of yoga practices or in non-basal states in particular yoga asanas or pranayamas, has now been considered. It is also of interest to have various measurements pertaining to the possible limits of air movement.

C.3 Vital Capacity

Vital capacity is that amount of air which a person can expire after a maximal inspiration. Thus, vital capacity is the total amount of air that can be moved into and out of the lungs in a breath. An average value for vital capacity is 4.5 liters. Several studies support the statement that vital capacity is increased after a period of hatha yoga. (See Figures 3.35 - 3.39.) The hatha yoga included asanas and pranayama in each study. The differences attributed to the yoga practice in each study are statistically significant. In Udupa's study[38] the average increase in vital capacity was .6 liters after 3 months and .9 liters after 6 months of hatha yoga. In Dhanaraj's study[39] the average increase was .5 liters after 6 weeks of hatha yoga; after a six-week period of detraining, this vital capacity increase was maintained. A group practicing the 5BX Program showed a .4 liter increase after 6 weeks. While Gopal's study[40] did not provide a value for the change in vital capacity, it did show that a group which was trained for 6 months in hatha yoga had an average vital capacity .9 liters greater than a group of comparable age which regularly engaged in light physical exercise such as long walks and games. Moses[41] found that vital capacity was significantly increased ($p < .01$) after 10 weeks of hatha yoga class for one group, compared to 10 weeks of physical exercise classes for a control group.

Bhole[42] measured vital capacity for 24 male experimental subjects and 24 male control subjects before and after a three-week summer course in yoga. The daily twelve-hour yoga practice session included 20 yoga postures and *shavasana* (corpse posture); 2 breathing practices, namely *ujjayi* and *kapalabhati* (skull-shining); and *agnisara, nauli* and *uddiyana-bandha* (abdominal lock). The experimental (yoga) group showed a statistically significant ($p < .001$) change in vital capacity, the increase amounting to about 4.2% (see Figure 3.39). The control group showed an insignificant change in vital capacity over the three-week period;

the initial values for vital capacity between the control group
and the experimental group did not differ significantly.

Udupa[43] further noted that vital capacity, when measured
after the physical stress of fast running, fell below its normal
value by an amount that was significantly less after 3 and 6
months of yoga training than initially. (See Figure 3.40.)

Although normally measured when a subject is upright,
vital capacity can be measured with the body in other positions.
Rao[44] found (see Figure 3.41) that vital capacity was less when
subjects practiced *shirshasana* (headstand) than when they were
standing; the difference was statistically significant ($p < .05$).

Two studies have noted certain other respiratory capacities.
Rao[45] found that inspiratory capacity (the amount of air that can
be drawn into the lungs after a normal expiration) and inspiratory
reserve volume (inspiratory capacity minus tidal volume) were
less in *shirshasana* (headstand) and in the erect standing position
than in the horizontal supine position. (See Figures 3.42 and
3.43.) Expiratory reserve volume (the quantity of air which,
after a normal expiration, it is possible to expel by further effort)
was much greater in the erect standing position than in *shirshasana* and in the horizontal supine position. (See Figure 3.44.)
Average differences in residual volume (the amount of air left in
the lungs after a maximal expiration) were found to be not statistically significant among the horizontal supine position, the erect
standing position, and *shirshasana*. (See Figure 3.45.) The functional reserve capacity (expiratory reserve volume plus residual
volume) was greater by a significant difference in the erect
standing position and in *shirshasana* than in the horizontal supine
position. (See Figure 3.46.) Differences in total lung capacity
(vital capacity plus residual volume) among the various positions
were not significant. (See Figure 3.47.) Differences between a
group trained in yoga and a group that was untrained in yoga and
engaged regularly in light physical exercise were not found by
Gopal[46] to be statistically significant for maximum breathing

capacity, timed vital capacity or maximum expiratory pressure. (See Figures 3.48, 3.49 and 3.50.)

D. Gaseous Transfer

The composition of inspired air is different from that of expired air. Inspired air is richer in oxygen and poorer in carbon dioxide and water vapor than expired air. Therefore, oxygen is used and carbon dioxide and water produced by the body in its activities. Providing fresh supplies of oxygen and removing carbon dioxide are seen as major functions of the respiratory activity. We will consider how several yoga practices and programs have been noted to affect oxygen absorption and carbon dioxide elimination.

Only 2 studies to date have considered the effect of a period of yoga practice on the basal metabolic rate. Basal metabolic rate is the rate at which oxygen is consumed when a person is resting in a supine position; the measurement should be made several hours after a meal so that digestive processes will be minimal. One study, by Dhanaraj,[47] measured the basal metabolic rate for 17 male college students before and after 6 weeks of practice of hatha yoga. The daily practice time was about 15 minutes and included 5 asanas and a pranayama practice. When expressed in terms of the percentage deviation from normal values for subjects of the same age and size, basal average metabolic rate was about .3% below the normal before and 5.3% above the normal after the yoga training. (See Figure 3.51.) Although the before-after difference is statistically significant ($p < .05$), the results are not of a magnitude to indicate excessively high metabolic rate after the yoga training. After a six-week de-training period, the basal metabolic rate had decreased slightly to 4.3% above normal. As regards respiratory quotient, which is defined as carbon dioxide output divided by oxygen intake, a normal value in basal state is .8, and in this experiment, the respiratory quotient was measured at .82 before and .81 after the yoga training; the difference was not statistically significant. (See Figure 3.52.)

The level of oxygen consumption in the basal state is viewed by physiologists to be related to the level of thyroid gland functioning. Dhanaraj, in fact, found an increase in the blood level of thyroxine, the principal thyroid hormone. (See Figure 4.1.) Included in the asanas practiced by his subjects were *sarvangasana* (shoulder stand) and *halasana* (plow posture). As was remarked in the previous chapter, *sarvangasana* (shoulder stand) and *halasana* (plow posture) increase the flow of blood through the thyroid gland. A study by Rangan[48] supports the statement that basal metabolic rate is increased by the practice of *sarvangasana* and *halasana*. Twelve physical education students performed the 2 asanas for 6 weeks, while 11 others served as a control group. Basal oxygen consumption was measured before and after the 6 weeks for all subjects, and the results were expressed in energy units of calories per hour and divided by body surface area to correct for size differences among subjects. The final basal metabolic rate was greater than the initial rate for both groups; only for the yoga group, however, was the difference statistically significant ($p < .05$). (See Figure 3.53.) This result suggests the need for further study to investigate the effect of practice of the shoulder stand and the plow posture in cases of hyperthyroidism and hypothyroidism to determine if the practices would lead to normalizing of functioning in all cases.

When the body is not resting but is engaging in physical activity, its consumption of oxygen increases. Oxygen consumption during vigorous exertion may be 50 times that of the basal state. The maximal oxygen consumption for the yoga group, 5BX group and control group was calculated by Dhanaraj from physical work capacity measurements according to certain accepted physiological procedures. It was found that while the average maximal oxygen consumption was greater after 6 weeks of practice than before, for both the yoga group and the 5BX group, the difference was highly significant ($p < .001$) for the 5BX group but not statistically significant for the yoga group. (See Figure 3.54.)

Salgar[49] determined the effect that the meditative posture *padmasana* (lotus posture) has on muscular efficiency. For this purpose he used 3 groups—one group consisted of 16 students who did no exercise or had a very low exercise level of any kind, a second group consisted of 10 subjects who had practiced *padmasana* for 40 minutes daily during the 6 months before the test, and a third group consisted of 12 subjects who had regularly performed such resistance exercises as lifting weights and using spring expanders during the 6 months before the test. The test consisted of pedalling a bicycle ergometer at 2 levels of workload, 100 kilogram meters per minute and 200 kilogram meters per minute, the first level being considered mild exercise and the second level being considered moderate exercise. Oxygen consumption was measured during a resting period and during the second half of a 10-minute exercise period on the ergometer. From these two measurements the amount of oxygen consumed during the exercise was calculated and a percent muscular efficiency, involving a ratio of the work level divided by the oxygen consumed, was computed.

The differences in average muscular efficiency between the yoga group and the non-exercise group, and between the yoga group and the conventional exercise group, were statistically significant ($p < .01$) at both the low level and the high level of exercise. (See Figure 3.55.) At both exercise levels the muscular efficiency of the yoga group was higher than that of the non-exercise group. The comparison between muscular efficiencies of the yoga group and the conventional exercise group, however, differed for the 2 exercise levels: the yoga group was more efficient at the low exercise level, whereas the conventional exercise group was more efficient at the high exercise level. Again the inter-group differences were significant statistically. Salgar suggests that yoga exercise is useful in increasing work efficiency in low-level exercise. This finding might be considered to have an implication for business management where there is a desire for a physical culture that will be useful for higher efficiency in clerical work. The validity of this implication should be further investi- gated in studies which involve other aspects of yoga than only asana *(padmasana)*, and which provide controls for initial inter- group differences in muscular efficiency.

Now that some long-term effects of repeated practice of yoga on oxygen consumption have been considered, it will be of interest to consider short-term effects of individual hatha yoga practices. The practices for which some evidence is available are *shavasana* (corpse posture), *padmasana* (lotus posture), *shirshasana* (headstand) and certain breathing practices.

Dhanaraj[50] determined the metabolic rate during *shavas- ana* (corpse posture). Seven subjects, who had trained for 6 weeks in a hatha yoga program which included *shavasana*, were measured for oxygen consumption rate after 15 minutes of sitting at rest in a chair and then after 15 minutes of *shavasana* relaxation. (See Figure 3.56.) There was a decrease from 269.6 to 241.9 ml./min. in the oxygen consumption. This 10.3% drop was greater than that of 3.5% seen in a group of 7 untrained subjects who rested in supine position for 15 minutes. The difference between pre- and post-treatment means in oxygen consumption for both groups was statistically significant ($p < .002$), as was the difference in post- treatment means between the 2 groups.

In unpublished data referred to by Salgar,[51] there was found during the practice of *padmasana* (lotus posture) an increase in oxygen consumption, in some cases by as much as 100 ml./min. According to Salgar, these figures suggest that *padmasana* is a mild form of exercise. When oxygen consumption is measured during meditative or pranayamic breathing exercises with subjects sitting in *padmasana*, perhaps this result, if confirmed by other experimenters, should be taken into account in interpreting the results.

As part of a study of *shirshasana* (headstand), Rao[52] determined the metabolic cost of this posture in comparison with other body positions. (See Figure 3.57.) Rao found that for his 6 subjects the mean metabolic rate was 200 ml. of oxygen per minute in the horizontal supine position. The erect standing position resulted in a usage of 227 ml./min. of oxygen, or 14.1% more than the oxygen utilization in the horizontal supine position. During *shirshasana* (headstand) there resulted a mean oxygen utilization of 336 ml./min., or an increase of 48% over that in the erect standing position and 69% over that in the horizontal supine position. According to one scheme for classifying different forms of work, *shirshasana* (headstand) would, from these data, be classified as light muscular exercise.

To determine the effect on oxygen utilization of an inverted posture without the interference of extra muscular activity, Rao measured the oxygen consumption of one subject who was suspended from a rope with the rope tied around the ankles. It was found in this case that the oxygen usage was 300 ml./min., or 30% more than the value in the erect standing position. Still, it is not clear why the metabolic cost of *shirshasana* (headstand) should be any greater than that of standing upright. This result suggests the need to determine the oxygen utilization required for *shirshasana* by those who are expert in hatha yoga. One might conjecture that for such subjects oxygen utilization in *shirshasana* would be the same as in standing upright. Indeed, Swami Kuvala-yananda[53] asserted that once *shirshasana* is mastered, the posture is no more difficult than standing on the legs.

Next, we consider the study made by Miles[54] on breathing exercises of *ujjayi*, *kapalabhati* (skull-shining) and *bhastrika* (bellows). Briefly, what Miles found was that the oxygen requirements in each of the breathing patterns tested exceeded the pre-experimental and post-experimental requirements of normal breathing in the same seated position. The accompanying figure (see Figure 3.58) summarizes measurements from 5 experiments for each of the 3 breathing exercises. In addition to the pre-experimental period there appears a mean value for both the first half and the second half of the experimental period, this peculiarity in the data having been made necessary by a limitation in the oxygen supply of the measuring device. The post-experimental period was designed to examine any after-effects, and was divided into 2 five-minute periods. The basal metabolic rate of the subject was tested to be 210 ml. of oxygen per minute.

In the *ujjayi* data the mean duration of the *ujjayi* period was 22 minutes. In the pre-normal period the oxygen consumption was 196 ml./min. In the first half of the *ujjayi* period this oxygen consumption increased by 18%. In the second half the oxygen consumption was increased by 32% over the pre-normal. The post-normal oxygen consumption was about 5% over the pre-normal.

In the *kapalabhati* (skull-shining) data, oxygen consumption increased in the first half of the experimental period by 10% over the pre-normal value of 198 ml./min. and in the second half by 14% over the pre-normal value. The post-normal oxygen consumption was about 3% lower than the pre-normal oxygen consumption.

In the *bhastrika* (bellows) data the pre-normal consumption was about 196 ml./min.; oxygen consumption was 17% greater than the pre-normal value in the first half of the *bhastrika* period and 20% greater than the pre-normal value in the second half of the *bhastrika* period. The oxygen consumption after the *bhastrika* period averaged about 3% below the pre-normal value in the first 5 minutes and 7% below pre-normal in the second 5 minutes.

Although an increase in oxygen consumption was noted in each breathing exercise, this increase was less in the *kapalabhati* (skull-shining) than in the *ujjayi* periods, and the average increase in oxygen consumption in the *bhastrika* (bellows) periods was between those of the *kapalabhati* and *ujjayi* periods. This result is consistent with the fact that *bhastrika*, as practiced by Miles's subject, was composed of interpositions of *ujjayi* periods and *kapalabhati* periods of breathing. It appears that the *kapalabhati* period of breathing, as evidenced in both *kapalabhati* alone and the *bhastrika* exercise, causes a subsequent slight decrease in oxygen consumption over the pre-normal period. Another factor of some interest is that the pre-normal oxygen consumption, when the subject was sitting in preparation for one of the breathing exercises and was breathing normally, averaged about 196 ml./min. and ranged from 185 ml./min. to 209 ml./min.—all of which are lower than the subject's reported basal metabolic rate of 210 ml./min. The general increase in oxygen consumption during the breathing exercises is explained by Miles as due to the control exerted over the respiratory muscles and the concomitant continuous overriding of stimuli from the respiratory centers of the nervous system.

Rao's study[55] of a subject practicing *ujjayi* produced results essentially in agreement with those of Miles. (See Figures 3.59 and 3.60.) Metabolic cost of *ujjayi* was 7.7% when it was practiced at a low altitude (520 meters) and 9.9% at a high altitude (3800 meters). These increases (7.7% and 9.9%) are less than the increase of 32% reported by Miles. One difference between the experiments conducted by Miles and Rao is the length of the *ujjayi* period; Miles's subject practiced *ujjayi* for about 20 minutes, Rao's for about 10 minutes. The oxygen consumption when *ujjayi* was practiced by Rao's subject at the higher altitude was 16% more than when the subject practiced *ujjayi* at the lower altitude.

Swami Kuvalayananda[56] ascertained that the carbon dioxide concentration of alveolar air after 2 minutes of *kapalabhati* (skull-shining) or after 5 minutes of *kapalabhati* was on the average almost identical with the carbon dioxide concentration of alveolar air after normal breathing. This study was undertaken to investigate the following chain of reasoning. First, it is generally believed, asserted Swami Kuvalayananda, that breath retention is increased if the practice of *kapalabhati* immediately precedes the attempt to hold the breath. Secondly, it is thought that the level of alveolar carbon dioxide would be inversely related to the length of breath holding time. Thus, it might have been thought that after a period of *kapalabhati* the carbon dioxide content of the alveolar air would be less than after normal breathing. The data obtained did not confirm this line of reasoning.

Swami Kuvalayananda[57] investigated the relation between oxygen absorption and carbon dioxide elimination and two aspects of yogic breathing. Two aspects of pranayama exercises are retention of breath and increased duration of the respiratory cycle. These modifications are made within a framework of maintaining certain ratios among the durations of inspiration, retention and expiration. Subjects performed 2 rounds of breathing in which certain counts for inspiration-retention-expiration were observed. (See Figures 3.61-3.64.) At the end of each round, expired air was collected and analyzed to determine volume percentage of oxygen absorption and carbon dioxide elimination. Data presented in Figures 3.61, 3.62, 3.63 and 3.64 are averages of measurements, 2 from each of 5 subjects. Figures 3.61 and 3.63 show that in general the volume percentage of oxygen absorption or carbon dioxide elimination increases as the total duration of the respiratory cycle increases. When, however, the volume percentage of gas is divided by the duration of the respiratory cycle, it is found that there is less oxygen absorption and carbon dioxide elimination per unit time when the duration of the respiratory cycle is increased. (See Figures 3.62 and 3.64.) Also, for a given length of respiratory cycle, the gaseous exchange per unit time is approximately the same whether or not retention of the breath constitutes part of the cycle. Swami Kuvalayananda contended that the value of increased duration of the respiratory cycle in pranayama, as well as the value of retention, is the preparation of the respiratory system for superior functioning throughout the day, rather than for their immediate efficiency in utilizing oxygen or releasing carbon dioxide.

Finally, in this section on gaseous transfer we consider certain data from the various confinement experiments. H. V. G. Rao's report [58] on an experienced student of hatha yoga (Yogi Ramananda of Mysore) who remained in a partially air-tight compartment for a nine-hour period indicated that the carbon dioxide and the oxygen content of the air in the pit was 3.8% at the end of the nine-hour session; after the two-hour confinement proportions of carbon dioxide and oxygen content in the pit were 1.34% and 18.79%, respectively. An expected amount of carbon dioxide in the pit could, on the basis of assumptions about the size and airtightness of the pit, be derived for any given average metabolic rate of the subject. The authors calculated that metabolic rate determined by a ventilation of 1 liter per minute would have to be assumed to account for the measured final carbon dioxide content of the compartment. A normal value for minute ventilation is 8 liters per minute.

Ballentine and Gibbons[59] reported gas analysis in a study of Yogi Ramananda during confinement in a sealed oxygen tent. (See Figure 3.65.) At the thirty-third minute of confinement, when the subject signalled to be released, the percentage of oxygen present was 12.8 and of carbon dioxide present was 7.14.

In the study by Karambelkar[60] it was found that oxygen consumption of 4 subjects had a smaller value while they were in the air-tight compartment than had been predicted on the basis of basal oxygen consumption for the individual subjects. It was further found that for those subjects with training in pranayama, the reduction in oxygen consumption while in the pit was less than for those with no training in pranayama, the differences being most noticeable as the percentages of carbon dioxide in the pit increased. Experiments with rats have indicated that a high percentage (such as 10%) of carbon dioxide in air will decrease oxygen consumption by 25%. These data suggest that in humans as well the oxygen consumption will be decreased by increasing ambient carbon dioxide content. The fact that this effect is much less pronounced in those experienced in pranayama indicates that the pranayama practice provides an acclimatization in such subjects to higher carbon dioxide content. The retention aspect of the pranayama exercises is suggested as a key feature in this carbon dioxide acclimatization process, since a high alveolar carbon dioxide content would be maintained during the retention phase.

During the confinement experiment conducted by Anand, the subject trained in yoga demonstrated less oxygen consumption than in basal state.[61]   In a ten-hour confinement, the average rate of oxygen consumption throughout the period was 13.3 liters per hour, in comparison to a basal oxygen requirement for the subject of 19.5 liters per hour. In one instance during the confinement, oxygen consumption was down as low as 10 liters per hour, and throughout the period it remained less than the subject's basal rate of utilization.

·4·

Endocrine and Nervous System Responses to Hatha Yoga

It is often asserted that the endocrine system and nervous system are toned or stimulated by hatha yoga practices. Indeed, attention to the well-being of these physiological systems is a feature that distinguishes hatha yoga from most systems of physical culture. The effects seem to arise in at least 2 different ways. First, local increases in blood circulation are brought about in the regions of the endocrine glands and nerve plexuses. This result may be accomplished by various asanas. For example, gravitational effects tend to increase circulation in the thyroid gland during *sarvangasana* (shoulder stand). Contraction of lumbo-sacral musculature in, for example, *bhujangasana* (cobra posture) would increase circulation to the plexus of that region; pressure by the elbows during *mayurasana* (peacock posture) would increase circulation in the region of the celiac, or solar, plexus. A second way in which endocrine-nervous system effects may arise occurs during pranayama. Prana is not readily identifiable with any physiologically defined entity or process; its

realm of activity and influence is considered by yogis to be different from the realm in which physiological activities occur. Nevertheless, the practices of pranayama, in which we include the
relaxation processes involving the manipulations of the breathing
system, are experienced as having major effects on the nervous
system.

Our purpose in this chapter will be to describe data which
pertain in a fairly direct manner to the endocrine and nervous
systems. Since these 2 systems control other systems of the
body, many of the results presented in previous chapters give
indirect information on the effects on these systems. Although
some authors have engaged in speculation as to why this or that
event occurred, we will for the most part forego such speculation
as the amount of factual information in these areas is so meager.

A. Secretory Products

There are 4 studies—one by Dhanaraj, two by Udupa, and
one by Karambelkar—which have considered changes in certain
endocrine products as a result of a daily period of hatha yoga
practices.

Dhanaraj[1] tested for the level of thyroxine in the blood
before and after 6 weeks of hatha yoga practice by a group of 17
male subjects. Thyroxine is considered to be the most important
hormone produced by the thyroid gland. In normal human serum
the amount of thyroxine ranges from 4 to 8 mg. per 100 ml.
Dhanaraj found that the average amount of thyroxine was greater
after 6 weeks of hatha yoga than before; a small decrease was
seen after 6 weeks of detraining in the group tested. (See Figure
4.1.) Small thyroxine decrements were noted after 6 weeks of
practice of the 5BX Program by a second group and after 6 weeks
in a control group. Of these differences, only the pre- and post-
treatment differences for the yoga group were found to be
statistically significant ($p < .05$). All average values were within the

normal range stated above.

The pair of adrenal glands, one atop each kidney, consists of 2 developmentally and functionally distinct endocrine glands, the adrenal medulla and the adrenal cortex. The adrenal medulla secretes the catecholamines, epinephrine and norepinephrine. Catecholamines tend to increase blood pressure, stimulate the nervous system, cause increased heat production and elevate the level of blood sugar. In the 2 studies conducted by Udupa, he reported a greater amount of catecholamines after than before periods of hatha yoga practice. (See Figures 4.2 and 4.3.) In one case,[2] the average measure of urinary catecholamines was changed by a statistically significant amount ($p < .05$) after 6 months of hatha yoga practice by 12 young adult males. (Specifically, what was reported was an increase in VMA, vanilly mandelic acid, a breakdown product of epinephrine.) In another case,[3] each of 4 subjects showed an increase in the level of plasma catecholamines after 3 months of either yoga practice or *suryanamaskar* (sun salutation). Three of these subjects showed an increase in blood histaminase as well. (See Figure 4.4.) Histaminase is an enzyme that breaks down histamine, which is involved in allergic reactions and causes vasodilatation.

The adrenal cortex produces a variety of hormones, which are chemically classified as steroids. Effects of the adrenal cortical hormones include elevating blood sugar, providing resistance to various stresses (bleeding, trauma, high altitude, temperature extremes, infection) and preventing allergic responses by inhibiting the production and secretion of histamine. Three of 4 subjects studied by Udupa[4] showed decreases in the level of plasma cortisol, one of the steroid hormones of the adrenal cortex, after 3 months of either yoga practice or *suryanamaskar* (sun salutation); the subject practicing *shirshasana* (headstand) and *mayurasana* (peacock posture) over this period showed an increase in plasma cortisol. (See Figure 4.5.) In Udupa's study of 12 subjects, the group showed after 3 and 6 months of training in hatha yoga an average increase in the amount of total urinary 17-hydroxysteroids (see Figure 4.6); these are metabolites of cortisol and corticosterone, another adrenal cortical hormone. The differences between the initial value and the value after 3 and 6 months were statistically significant (p < .1). The level of urinary production of 17-ketosteroids (derived from hormones produced by the adrenal cortex and testis) decreased after 3 months of hatha yoga but had increased after 3 more months; (see Figure 4.7) the difference between the initial and 3-month levels was statistically significant (p<.05).

Karambelkar[5] considered the level of uropepsin before and after 19 subjects were trained for 3 weeks in 20 asanas. Uropepsin is a urinary component that breaks down proteins; it is of gastric origin. The study showed (see Figure 4.8) that the uropepsin level decreased from 19.9 units per hour to 11.4 units per hour for the treatment group, whereas in a control group the decrease was found to be from 16.1 to 14. The yoga group's decrease was statistically significant (p < .001). The separate data for the 5 females among the 18 experimental subjects showed a non-significant decrease from 14 to 7.2 units. This result could, Karambelkar suggested, be due to the small size of the experimental group of females and also to the initially lower uropepsin levels among females as compared to males. The mean decrease for the 15 males in the experimental subjects was from 22.2 to 13 units of uropepsin per hour. Karambelkar asserted that there has been postulated a close relationship between the excretion of uropepsin and adrenal cortical function. If such a relationship does hold, then the preceding may be viewed as evidence of decreased adrenal cortical activity.

The only results found by Udupa[6] that remain to be described concern acetylcholine and cholinesterase, levels for both of which decreased after 3 months of either yoga practice or *suryanamaskar* (sun salutation) by 4 subjects. (See Figures 4.9 and 4.10.) Acetylcholine functions as the chemical transmitter of electrical impulses at most nerve-nerve and nerve-muscle junctions; it is also a potent vasodilator. Cholinesterase is an enzyme that deactivates acetycholine once its transmission function is performed. Acetylcholine and cholinesterase levels were also determined by Udupa[7] initially and after 3 and 6 months of daily hatha yoga practice by 12 young males (the same group which was discussed two paragraphs above). (See Figures 4.11 and 4.12.) After three months the mean value for plasma acetylcholine had decreased ($p < .1$), as had that for serum cholinesterase ($p < .05$). A further decrease in acetylcholine level was seen after 6 months ($p < .01$ when compared with the initial value by a t-test), while a slight increase in cholinesterase was seen after 6 months (the comparison with the initial level was still statistically significant.)

B. Autonomic Balance

The autonomic nervous system is defined functionally as that portion of the nervous system which sends efferent fibers to the smooth muscles and the glands of the body. The autonomic nervous system is divided along anatomical lines into the sympathetic and parasympathetic nervous systems. Since the autonomic nervous system is concerned with all the visceral actions in the body, and since parasympathetic and sympathetic fibers often interact in many visceral organs in the body, a comparison of sympathetic and parasympathetic functions can be made by determining activity levels for various visceral functions. Wenger developed a means of using several such physiological variables to arrive at a number called the "autonomic balance" of an individual.

Gharote[8] determined the autonomic balance score for a control group and an experimental group of adolescent males (mean age 15 years). The experimental group underwent 2 months of a program including training in the following yoga

practices: *bhujangasana* (cobra posture), *ardha-shalabhasana*
(half-locust posture), *dhanurasana* (bow posture), *viparitakarani*
(inverted action), *sarvangasana* (shoulder stand), *matsyasana*
(fish posture), *halasana* (plough posture), *chakrasana* (wheel
posture), *vakrasana* (twisted posture), *utkatasana* (squatting
pose), *vrikshasana* (tree posture), *paschimottanasana* (posterior
stretching posture), *vajrasana* (supine pelvic posture), *mayurasana*
(peacock posture) *uddiyana-bandha* (abdominal lock), *ujjayi*,
and *shavasana* (corpse posture). The two groups were paired
according to scores on the McCurdy Larson Organic Efficiency
Test.

The autonomic balance score is a normally distributed
variable with an average value of 69, according to studies by
Wenger. The initial values in the control group and experimental
group studied by Gharote were 62.25 and 64.64, respectively.
(See Figure 4.13.) After the 2 months period, the value of autonomic balance for the control group was 67.77, and that for the
experimental group was 78.07. The difference in final scores
was statistically significant (p < .01). According to Wenger, above
average scores indicate relatively higher parasympathetic function
and below average scores indicate relatively higher sympathetic
function. Gharote's experiment thus implies that there is an increase in the direction of parasympathetic function after 2
months' practice of yoga. A subsequent two-month period, in
which the experimental group was instructed to discontinue
practicing yoga, resulted in a decrease of 3.49 in the group's
autonomic balance score; statistically this was not a significant
change. Thus, the change in autonomic balance was retained
even when the practice of yoga was discontinued for 2 months.

The physiological factors from which the autonomic
balance score was computed in Gharote's study are: salivary
output, sublingual temperature, palmar conductance, log conductance change, volar conductance, diastolic blood pressure and
heart period.   Conductance measurements have been reported

separately in yoga studies. Conductance is a measure of the ease with which electric current can pass through a given material; it is the reciprocal of the electrical resistance. Palmar conductance measures the conductance between electrodes placed on the palm of the hand, while volar conductance measures that between electrodes placed on the sole of the foot. Log conductance change refers to the logarithmic difference between conductance in two conditions, tension followed by relaxation. Conductance, or resistance, is considered by psychophysiologists to be an indirect measurement sensitive to sweating; lower values of conductance correlate with lower amounts of skin moisture.

Wenger[9] conducted studies of autonomic function in various practitioners of yoga. He found that values for palmar conductance and log conductance change were very low among a group of serious yoga students in comparison with norms determined from various United States subjects. He considered these findings to be evidence that the yoga students had acquired an ability to relax voluntarily. When these subjects practiced *shavasana* (corpse posture) there was found to be a slight decrease in palmar conductance. (See Figure 4.14.) When the subjects practiced any of various breathing exercises (*ujjayi*, *bhastrika* [bellows] *kapalabhati* [skull-shining] or the non-yogic exercise of hyperventilation), increases in palmar conductance were found. (See Figures 4.15 and 4.16.)

V. Pratap[10] considered palmar conductance measurements in response to various stimuli. The subjects, who all had practiced yoga for at least a year, first relaxed against a support in a reclining position; later they were asked to sit erect in a meditative posture and relax. Subjects were instructed to maintain stability in the posture, whether reclining or erect. During each of these conditions the subjects were presented with various stresses—a flood lamp illuminated nearby for a few seconds; an ice bag placed on the thigh; a mental arithmetic problem posed for solution; and a loud noise made nearby. The response levels of certain physiological parameters prior to and during the presentation of these stressors were noted. In each case, average response level for palmar conductance was less when the subjects were in the erect yogic posture. The response level and its percentage change, for the variables of respiratory rate and percent time of occipital alpha, were generally less in the yogic condition than in the non-yogic condition.

In confinement experiments, Karambelkar[11] found the skin resistance to be constant in the confinement period until the ambient carbon dioxide concentration reached the level of about 5%, at which time skin resistance increased significantly. This was found to be true independently of the amount of practice in yoga of the person confined.

C. EEG

EEG measurements have played little part to date in the scientific studies of hatha yoga. We have elsewhere in this consideration of hatha yoga discussed various physiological characteristics of a subject, studied by Anand,[12] during a ten-hour confinement period. An EEG record, with multiple bipolar leads, was made before and at several intervals during the confinement. Prior to and soon after confinement, there was a dominant alpha rhythm. Soon this was replaced by a low voltage high frequency activity which, except for occasional runs of prominent alpha or hump activity (associated with drowsiness), was characteristic of the subject's EEG throughout the confinement. No delta waves (associated with deep sleep) were recorded.

The EEG of Yogi Ramananda during confinement experiments was recorded by Rao[13] to be similar to the subject's normal resting EEG: there was a regular alpha rhythm, the subject remained alert throughout the confinement periods and he showed no tendency toward drowsiness or sleep. The occipital EEG of this subject during a confinement experiment conducted by

Ballentine and Gibbons [14] showed a gradual slight slowing of prominent alpha frequency from 9-10 Hz. initially to 8 Hz. at the experiment's termination.

Hirai[15] briefly instructed an individual with no Zen experience in the breath-count breathing control practice of Zen. When the subject sat, with eyes open, and practiced this technique, short trains (1-2 seconds) of alpha waves were seen amid the predominant beta wave activity.

Two studies, one by J. V. Hardt and one by B. Timmons and colleagues, associated EEG features with certain aspects of breathing which may be relevant to studies of yoga, although in neither case were the subjects said to be students of yoga.

In Hardt's study[16] percent time of EEG alpha over a ten-minute period of breathing practice was compared with a subject's baseline percent time of alpha. Each subject was taught one of 3 types of breathing. First, there was a slow breathing technique, modeled on a yoga breathing technique, in which the subject was to inhale, hold, and exhale, with equal time allotted to each phase. Second, this slow breathing was accompanied by audio feedback of the subject's amplified breathing sounds. (This feedback of breath sounds may be analogous in effect to paying attention to the sensations of the breath entering and leaving the nostrils.) Third, there was fast, shallow breathing. There was much greater increase in alpha level over baseline alpha during the slow breathing than during the fast breathing; adding feedback of breath sounds resulted in a small further increase in alpha level over baseline.

Timmons[17] considered the relation between EEG changes and changes in breathing patterns during waking and sleep states. Eleven subjects with no particular experience in yoga or other meditative systems were asked to recline in a supine position and were instructed to relax and go to sleep. During this period the EEG was recorded in a mono-polar fashion (left-central/left-occipital). Eye movements were measured, and respiratory movements of the thorax and the abdomen were monitored by separate strain gauges.

The initial waking state EEG pattern was predominantly alpha; it was accompanied in 10 subjects by abdominal dominant breathing. (See Figure 4.17.) In the period of drowsiness and Stage 1 sleep, abdominal breathing amplitude tended to decrease and thoracic amplitude to increase; for all subjects there were instants of equality between abdominal and thoracic breath amplitudes. In 9 subjects, thoracic dominant breathing occurred in Stage 1 sleep or in Stage 2 sleep.

Increases and decreases in abdominal amplitude, but not thoracic amplitude, of breathing correlated with EEG transitions in or out of alpha. (See Figure 4.18.) A reduction of abdominal amplitude occurred in 93% of the EEG transitions in which alpha disappeared from the record for a period of at least 10 seconds (alpha-theta transition). An increase in abdominal amplitude occurred in 81% of the cases in which there was a return of alpha rhythm for at least 5 seconds (theta-alpha transition). Timmons suggested that since changes in consciousness, as defined by EEG parameters, are accompanied by changes in respiratory patterns, control of states of consciousness might be facilitated by controlling respiratory patterns. Such a viewpoint is found in yoga, Zen, and other meditative disciplines that utilize breathing techniques.

With the subjects in the waking state, the inspiratory phase of the abdominal cycle of breathing was longer than the expiratory phase, whereas in the drowsiness of Stage 1 sleep, the inspiratory and expiratory phases became approximately equal. This equality continued for most subjects who went further into Stage 2 sleep.

The thoracic cycle of breathing, because of its low amplitude and inconsistent nature, was not related to wakefulness. However, in those cases where the thoracic amplitude was greater than abdominal amplitude, the inspiratory phase was longer than the expiratory phase. Also, the wave form of inspiration and expiration was characteristically skewed, the expiratory phase showing a magnitude of deceleration greater than that of acceleration for the inspiratory phase.

Part II

Physiological Responses
to Meditation

·5·

General Physiological Responses to Meditation

A. Background

A.1 Description of Meditation

Hatha yoga, as viewed by the proponents of Raja Yoga, is preliminary and adjunctive to meditation. Meditation is a practice whereby the individual may accurately experience his own nature and that of the universe. As presented by Patanjali in the *Yoga Sutras*, it is the next-to-last in the series of 8 stages of yoga, the last 4 of which are as follows: *pratyahara* (withdrawal of the senses), *dharana* (concentration), *dhyana* (meditation) and *samadhi* (the superconscious state). The following paragraph, based on the chapters "What is Meditation?" and "Samadhi" from Swami Rama's *Lectures on Yoga*,[1] may serve as a summary of the process of moving through these 4 stages.

"Every time one meditates one reaches the state of

meditation only by systematically going through the six preliminary stages." First, mindfulness of the *yamas* (moral restraints) and *niyamas* (observances) helps the student establish within himself a harmonious mental background. Relaxed, the student "assumes a meditative posture which is steady and comfortable and ensures that the head, neck and trunk are erect and in one straight line . . . . Sitting in the meditative posture, the student practices such exercises of pranayama as *bhastrika* (bellows), which refreshes his air supply and makes the mind more alert and free from drowsiness," and *nadi shodhanam* (alternate nostril breathing), which strengthens and purifies the nervous system and calms the mind. Now, "the right and left breath are equalized, the breathing becomes deeper and more gentle." In the next step, *pratyahara*, the student mentally withdraws to his immediate spatio-temporal environment and mentally reaffirms, "I am not the body, I am not the senses. They are my instruments. I am not the mind. The mind is my subtler instrument. I am the *Atman*, the Infinite." Then, in *dhyana* (meditation), he "tries to make his mind one-pointed through voluntary attention and concentration." The object of concentration may be a visual or auditory image or some other object. Having concentrated the divergent activities of the conscious mind, the student's mind in *dhyana* (meditation) flows uninterruptedly toward the object of concentration. Thus "concentration leads to one-pointedness, and prolonged concentration leads to meditation." The one-pointed mind in meditation may then expand into the superconscious state of *samadhi*, in which the original objects of concentration and the mental observer of that object are no longer distinct but are identified.

A.2 Classification of Experiments on Meditation

Having read the preceding definitional statements on meditation, the reader should understand that the subjects of

scientific experiments on meditation have practiced meditation
according to the instructions of various schools and teachers. In
this section we classify the scientific investigations described in
Chapters 5 and 6 according to the meditative procedures which
the subjects followed.

The subjects studied by Anand, Gharote, Green, Swami
Kuvalayananda, and Wenger practiced meditation according to
the precepts of Raja Yoga as described in Section A.1 above.

The subjects studied by Das practiced meditation according
to the precepts of Kriya Yoga. This procedure was described by
Das as follows:

> In this technique, the Kundalini arrives at (or ascends to) the
> frontal region where the *ajana chakra* is located, showing it-
> self (or manifesting) as a light seen by the subject, whose eyes
> are closed, gaze fixed between the eyebrows; this light then
> becomes the object of contemplation (*bindu-dhyana*); it be-
> comes increasingly intense, vibrating and it dissolves in a million
> stars, in the midst of which one discerns the figure of his deity.[2]

The subjects studied by Banquet, F. M. Brown, Benson,
Dhanaraj, Jevning, Levander, Orme-Johnson, Pagano, Rieckert,
Schwartz and Wallace practiced meditation according to the
precepts of Transcendental Meditation. The technique of Transcendental Meditation has been defined as "turning the attention
inwards towards the subtler levels of a thought until the mind
transcends the experience of the subtlest state of the thought
and arrives at the source of the thought."[3]

The subjects studied by Hirai, Kasamatsu and Sugi practiced
meditation according to the precepts of *zazen*. Hirai explained
that *zazen* is the seated Zen meditation, and this system "consists
of three major parts: breath control, posture control, and mind
control . . . . The basic nature of *zazen* meditation is a dialogue
with the self: it provides a time of calm, undisturbed or distracted
by thoughts, in which the individual can listen to the voice that is
within."[4] The origin of the Japanese word *Zen* is the Sanskrit
word *dhyana*, which is, as we have seen, the word for meditation
in the system of Raja Yoga.

A.3 Organization of Part II

Since the activity of meditation is considered mental, and since mental events are considered by physiologists to be somehow related to events in the brain, and since EEG recording has been widely used as a technique to study brain activities, it is not surprising that many physiological studies of meditation have collected data on EEG activity in meditation. After the present chapter has dealt with all physiological variables other than the EEG, the next chapter will report on all the EEG research on meditation available at the present time.

B. Muscular System Responses to Meditation

From the point of view of the skeletal muscular system, meditational practices are traditionally static. An asana was considered by Patanjali in the *Yoga Sutras* to be a seated posture in which the body could be put most easily and comfortably while the mind practiced meditation. The meditative asanas mentioned in the *Yoga Sutras* are all variations of sitting cross-legged, with attention given to maintenance of the normal erect curvature of the spine.

A study was made by N. N. Das[5] of 7 subjects in India. During meditation (Kriya Yoga meditation) the subjects sat in the lotus posture. Electrodes were attached to the right and left quadriceps muscles of the legs and EMG readings were taken continuously during the meditative period. During most of the meditative period the EMG recorded zero activity of the quadriceps muscles.

The 12 experimental subjects studied by J. P. Banquet in the United States had practiced a meditational technique (Transcendental Meditation) for an average of 2 years. There was also a control group of 12 subjects who planned to learn meditation.[6] During the experiment the primary concern was EEG measurements, as it had been in the experiments by Das.

The subjects in Banquet's experiment were seated comfortably in chairs and they attended initially to maintaining the erectness and proper alignment of the head, neck and trunk.

In 6 of the 12 experimental subjects, the EMG was recorded using an electrode placed below the chin and linked to the ears as reference electrode. It was found in these subjects (EMG was not recorded for the other subjects) that the voltage of EMG activity became very low. It was also noticed that muscle artifacts which in the EEG records appear like "fast frequencies of large amplitude on the spectral arrays disappeared early during meditation." Frontal EEG electrodes can detect activity of small muscles that control eye movements. During the beginning of meditation, eye movements were found to become slow. In stages that were characterized by the subjects as "deep meditation" there were no eye movements. On occasions, reported by the subjects to coincide with kaleidoscopic visual activity, there were bursts of rapid eye movements of the type associated with dreaming.

Although muscular activity is slight during meditation, the capacity for voluntary muscular action was, in the case of the subjects studied by Banquet, found to remain. Next to a subject's hand was a set of 5 push-buttons which he was to use to classify internal experience into the following categories: body sensation, involuntary movement, visual imagery, deep meditation, or transcendence (deepest meditation). Even during stages reported in this push-button schema as transcendence, the voluntary muscle activity was available to do the recording. Some subjects were occasionally asked certain questions and they provided accurate verbal responses. This ability to utilize the voluntary skeletal musculature in the state termed "transcendence" by the subjects in Banquet's experiment is in significant contrast with other descriptions of meditative states in which there is no interaction with the environment.

C. Circulatory System Responses to Meditation

We now consider changes in the circulatory system attributed to meditation—first, regional alterations in blood flow. Wenger[7] measured various physiological changes occurring during meditation (Raja Yoga meditation) as performed in India by 4 yoga students (2 to 7 years' experience), and 4 older yogis. These were all residents of Kaivalyadhama. Average values were reported for measurements taken over four 2½ minute intervals: before meditation, after 5 minutes of meditation, in the middle of meditation and 10 minutes before the end of meditation; the period of meditation lasted about 50 minutes on the average. It was found that in the five-minute pre-meditation period the finger temperature of the students of yoga averaged about 31.5° C. After 5 minutes of meditation there was an average increase to 32° C. In the middle and towards the end of the meditation, finger temperature averaged less than 31° C. (See Figure 5.1.) For the older yogis, the finger temperature began before the meditation at about 30.3 degrees and increased by half a degree towards the end of the period of meditation. The initial values were much lower for the older yogis than for the young yoga students but the values late in the meditation were quite similar for the two groups. During *shavasana* (corpse posture), practiced by the yoga students, the finger temperatures averaged 1½ to 3°C. more than during the students' meditation. Wenger also measured finger blood volume changes plethysmographically during meditation. For the yoga students, the average finger pulse volume was slightly higher after meditation began but returned to the pre-meditation level at the middle and late stages of meditation. (See Figure 5.2.) For the older yogis, the situation was somewhat different, as the average pulse volume at the mid-meditation reading was almost 20% higher than that of the pre-meditation period. The finger pulse volume was greater initially for the older yogis than for the yoga students and, during meditation, changes were more pronounced for the older subjects.

H. Rieckert[8] measured plethysmographically the circulation of blood in the finger and forearm. Finger blood flow gives an indication of skin circulation, whereas forearm blood flow gives an indication of muscular circulation. It was found (see Figure 5.3) that during meditation (Transcendental Meditation) the circulation in the forearm increased significantly ($p < .01$), by as much as 300% in some individuals, whereas the finger circulation decreased slightly ($p < .1$). Rieckert contrasted these changes with changes that occurred in another group of subjects practicing autogenic training. For the group, finger circulation increased significantly ($p < .02$) whereas the forearm circulation increased to a less significant degree ($p < .05$).

V. L. Levander[9] measured, with a water plethysmograph, forearm blood flow before, during and after periods of either meditation (Transcendental Meditation) or rest in a group of 5 healthy male subjects. A small but significant ($p < .025$) average increase in forearm blood flow was found in the meditation period as compared to pre-meditation rest (see Figure 5.4). When the subjects continued to rest with eyes closed in a seated position instead of meditating, slight decrease (9%) was found in the forearm blood flow.

In his studies of meditation (Transcendental Meditation), R. K. Wallace [10] found no significant change in rectal temperature during meditation. (See Figure 5.5.) It had been conjectured that the meditative experience might in some ways be analagous to hibernation; but rectal temperature in animals during hibernation has been found to decrease significantly, so Wallace's data did not confirm the speculated analogy.

At this point, we will consider relations between blood pressure and meditation. Wenger [11] found that in younger yoga students during meditation both systolic and diastolic blood pressure readings were slightly greater towards the end of meditation than in the pre-meditation period. Similarly, for the older yogis differences between treatment and pre-treatment blood pressure readings were small. (See Figures 2.32.) All average blood pressure readings were greater for the older yogis in meditation than for the younger students in meditation, and still less for the younger students in *shavasana* relaxation.

Wallace[12] found a slight increase in average systolic and diastolic blood pressures from the pre-meditation period to the meditative period and from the meditative period to the post-meditation period; the differences were not statistically significant. (See Figure 5.6.)

Although subjects for the studies by Wenger and by Wallace were not considered to be hypertensive, Datey and Patel had, it may be recalled from Chapter 2, found that blood pressure decreased in hypertensive patients who practiced yoga relaxation. (See Figures 2.30-2.42.) The relaxation technique taught by Patel, moreover, included a meditative factor: mental repetition of a word of thought in synchrony with the respiratory rhythm. Although meditation was found to have no effect on the blood pressure of normotensive subjects, H. Benson [13] tested the hypothesis that meditation (Transcendental Meditation) decreases the blood pressure of hypertensive persons. In Benson's experiment, 14 subjects, during a control period before meditation had been learned, were measured to have average systolic blood pressure of 145.6 mm. Hg. After the meditative technique had been taught to the subjects and practiced by them for several weeks (20 weeks on the average), the subjects' average systolic blood pressure decreased to 135.0 mm. Hg. (See Figure 5.7.) These measurements were not taken during the periods of meditation but at random times during the day. The decrease was from the range of high blood pressure to that of normal blood pressure, and the change was found to be statistically significant ($p < .01$). Diastolic blood pressure measurements showed a decrease from 91.9 to 87.0 mm. Hg. after several weeks of practice in meditation; these changes in diastolic blood pressures were statistically significant ($p < .05$). Levels of antihypertensive medication were maintained without change throughout the experiment. Some subjects chose to stop the regular practice of meditation after they had shown some lowering of blood pressure. Within 4 weeks of this detraining in meditation the blood pressure had returned to initial hypertensive levels.

Next, let us discuss observations on heart rate during meditation. Most data suggest that heart rate decreases during the period of meditation. Wallace found in one study[14] that the heart rate of subjects during meditation decreased an average of 5 beats per minute. In another study[15] made by Wallace and his colleagues, heart rate decreased during meditation by 3 beats per minute from a pre-meditation rate of 70 beats per minute. This difference was found to be statistically significant ($p < .05$). After the period of meditation the heart rate resumed the average value of the pre-meditation period. (See Figure 5.8.)

Dhanaraj[16] made various physiological comparisons among meditation as practiced by 7 college students having some experience with Transcendental Meditation, *shavasana* (corpse posture) relaxation as practiced by 7 other college students, and simple supine rest as practiced by a control group. Experimental data were collected before and after fifteen-minute practice periods. He found a decrease in heart rate from 70 to 64.3 beats per minute in comparing post- and pre-meditation periods. This decrease of 6.7 beats per minute is less than the decrease of 9.5 beats per minute found by Dhanaraj in subjects practicing *shavasana* (corpse posture), but was greater than the 5.2 beats per minute found in control subjects relaxing in supine position. (See Figure 5.9.) The heart rate changes were statistically significant ($p < .02$) for each of the 3 groups.

In both older and younger yoga practitioners studied by Wenger [17] the heart rate increased by 1 or 2 beats per minute during meditation. (See Figure 5.10.) This increase was found to be slightly greater in the younger yoga students than in the older yogis.

Das[18] reported that in general there was very little variation in the cardiac rhythm during meditation. An exception to the general trend was observed in one subject during a period of meditation ending, according to the report, in *samadhi*. Before the meditation the heart rate was 85 beats per minute in this subject. During light meditation this increased to 90 beats per minute and during deep meditation and *samadhi* the increase was to 95 beats per minute. After meditation the heart rate dropped to 70 beats per minute. Das conjectured, on the basis of this observation, that the heart rate generally accelerates during *samadhi*.

T. Hirai[19] found that pulse rate was accelerated during *zazen* to between 80 and 100 beats per minute.

Very few studies have assayed blood composition during meditation. One such study made by Wallace [20] found no significant change in pH during meditation. (See Figure 5.11.) Wallace did find, however, a statistically significant change ($p < .005$) in blood lactate from an average value of 11.4 mg./100 ml. in the pre-meditation period to 8.0 mg./100 ml. during meditation; the post-meditation period showed a further decrease to 7.3 units of blood lactate (see Figure 5.12). Anaerobic metabolism in skeletal muscles is presumed to be a major source of lactate production. Therefore, decrease in blood lactate in meditation " might be explained by increased skeletal muscle blood flow with constant increased aerobic metabolism." High blood lactate levels have been associated with anxiety symptoms as well as with essential and renal hypertension.

In meditating Zen priests, Hirai[21] reported a decrease in the amount of lactic acid in the blood.

D. Respiratory System Responses to Meditation

The general experience of those who practice meditation is that there is a decrease in both rate and amplitude of respiration during meditation; this subjective observation has been confirmed in several different experiments.

Hirai[22] found that the breathing pattern was changed in

priests practicing *zazen*, decreasing to 4-5 per minute. The amplitude of abdominal breathing was greater than that of thoracic
breathing, and both amplitudes were greater than those seen in
normal breathing.

The young yoga students studied by Wenger [23] (see Figure
3.12) showed a drop after the first 5 minutes of meditation from
about 14 breaths per minute to 6 or 7, and an approximate constancy of this respiration rate during the rest of the meditative period.
This pattern contrasts with a decrease from about 26 breaths per
minute to about 9 breaths per minute during *shavasana* practiced
by the same yoga students. The older yogis measured by Wenger
showed an average breath rate before meditation of only about
6 breaths per minute. This dropped by 1 or 2 breaths per minute
early in the meditative period but later during meditation returned
to about 6 or 7 breaths per minute. These individuals, who had
been practicing meditation for many years, had perhaps an ambient
breath rate lower than those students who had practiced yoga for
only a few years, and their breath rate did not change during meditation to the degree seen in the less experienced yoga students.

Dhanaraj[24] reported moderate decrease from the initial
value in respiration rate measured after meditation (see Figure
3.11), after *shavasana* (corpse posture), and after supine rest (practiced by controls). The average differences between pre-treatment
and post-treatment means were statistically significant ($p < .005$)
for each group, but the post-treatment differences between the
groups were not statistically significant ($p < .2$).

Wallace [25] reported finding a significant decrease from 13
breaths per minute before meditation to 22 breaths per minute
during meditation ($p < .05$). (See Figure 5.13.)

In a subject studied by Allison, [26] at the onset of meditation (Transcendental Meditation) respiration rate dropped from the
range of 10 to 15 breaths per minute to the range of 4 to 6 breaths
per minute and did not increase above 8 breaths per minute during
meditation. At the end of meditation the breath rate rose again

to the pre-meditation level of 12 breaths per minute. The record shown by Allison is noticeable for the precipitate decrease of breath rate at the onset of meditation and the precipitate return to the pre-meditation level at the end of meditation.

In Allison's study the minute ventilation was indirectly studied during meditation. Near the nostrils and mouth of the subject were placed thermistors whose temperature change varied with the amount of respired air passing over them. The mean thermistor temperature was found to increase at the beginning of meditation, remain approximately constant during meditation and decrease at the end of meditation. The increase indicated that the volume of air crossing the externally heated thermistors was less, thereby cooling the thermistors less. Although the magnitude of minute ventilation was not determined directly, it could be inferred to have changed abruptly at both the onset and end of the meditation period.

Dhanaraj[27] reported that the average tidal volume was less in a post-meditation period than in a pre-meditation period. (See Figure 3.28.) He also reported a decrease of tidal volume in a group practicing *shavasana* (corpse posture) but an increase in tidal volume in a control group resting in a supine position. The differences in tidal volume were statistically significant ($p < .005$) for each group. The difference between the post-treatment levels for the meditation and *shavasana* groups was insignificant, while the control group's final breath rate was significantly higher ($p < .05$) than that of either of the other groups.

Wallace[28] found a significant change in minute ventilation ($p < .05$) from 6.08 litres per minute in a pre-control period to 5.4 during a period of meditation. (See Figure 5.14.) Consistent with the findings of Allison of rapid re-attainment of normal respiratory activity, Wallace found a post-meditation period ventilation of 5.94. Wallace stated elsewhere that during meditation the "observed decrease in total ventilation was caused by either decreased frequency of breath or tidal volume, varying from subject to subject."[29] (See also Figure 5.15.)

We will now consider the various components of gas exchange as they have been seen to be modified by meditation. In
all studies of meditation where oxygen consumption has been one
of the variables measured, the consumption of oxygen has been
found to decrease during meditation. Since this condition of
decreased metabolic activity during meditation has been found by
some studies to occur along with other physiological conditions (for
example, the EEG pattern) characteristic of wakefulness, some
authors have referred to "the" physiological state occurring during
meditation as a "wakeful hypometabolic physiologic state."[30] The
elicitation of these physiological changes is further viewed as a
hypothalamically integrated response, referred to by Benson as the
"relaxation response."[31] Meditation, Benson suggests, is only one
among many methods by which the relaxation response may be
evoked.

Dhanaraj[32] found a 15.5% drop in oxygen consumption after
15 minutes of meditation (see Figure 3.54). The pre-meditation
oxygen consumption level was 257 ml./min.; after 15 minutes of
meditation the oxygen consumption averaged 216.9 ml./min. This
decrease in oxygen consumption was compared to that of a group
of subjects practicing *shavasana* for 15 minutes. Compared to the
initial level, there was a 10.3% drop in oxygen consumption after
shavasana.   A control group resting in supine position for 15
minutes dropped 3.5% in oxygen consumption. Oxygen consumption among the three groups was significant statistically ($p < .001$)
when the differences between post-treatment means were compared.
The difference in means between pre-treatment and post-treatment
was statistically significant ($p < .002$) for each of the three groups.

Wallace (1970)[33] reported that average oxygen consumption
in pre-meditation rest was 244.4 cm³ /min. After 10 minutes of
meditation, the average oxygen consumption was 208.1; after 20
minutes of meditation it was 201.9; after 30 minutes of meditation
it was 200.8. After meditation, oxygen consumption rose to 233.1.
(See Figure 5.16.)   The decrease is about 20% overall during

meditation as compared to the pre-meditation period. The post-meditation value was measured after 15 minutes of resting following meditation and was close to the pre-meditation level. Wallace (1971) [34] reported in a study of 20 subjects a decrease from 251.2 ml/min. in pre-meditation to 211.4 ml./min. during meditation, a significant ($p<.005$) change of about 17% in oxygen consumption. (See Figure 5.17.) The oxygen consumption gradually increased after meditation to 242.1 ml./min.

Sugi [36] compared the energy consumption in 4 meditating Zen priests with their basal metabolic rate, and found that metabolic rate averaged 19% below basal metabolic rate during *zazen*. (See Figure 5.18.)

Gharote [36] measured the change in metabolic rate during meditation (Raja Yoga meditation) practiced by a subject who on other occasions had gone into a meditative state considered to be profound. (See Figure 5.19.) In this state the subject had evidenced non-responsiveness to external stimuli and diminution of EEG and ECG voltages. Oxygen consumption was reported for this subject in the units of calories per square meter per hour. The mean over 3 days of measurement of metabolic rate in sitting prior to meditation was 37.1, only .1 higher than the subject's basal metabolic rate. The mean during meditation was 29.67. This mean, formed from measurements taken at 15-minute intervals during meditation was less than the pre-meditation mean ($p < .5$). The metabolic rate as tested soon after meditation was 40.03, significantly different from the mean during meditation ($p<.01$). and, although greater, not significantly different from the pre-meditation period average. In agreement with data reported by Wallace (see Figure 5.16), the third (last) metabolic rate measurement during meditation had for this subject invariably the lowest value among those measurements taken during meditation. The percentage decrease in metabolic rate in this experiment was on the average 25%, somewhat more than that reported by Dhanaraj, Wallace and Sugi (see the preceding three paragraphs).

Meditation involves periods of prolonged sitting in one posture; although one might have expected the prolonged sitting to provide a metabolic rate higher than the basal rate, the metabolic rate during meditation is below the basal metabolic rate. (See Figure 5.16.) The rapidity with which the decreases in oxygen consumption occur in meditation surpasses that normally seen in oxygen consumption decreases in sleep, which normally vary from 10% to 20% below basal levels.

Some studies have measured the change in carbon dioxide elimination during meditation as well as the change in oxygen consumption. Wallace [37] reported that in the pre-meditation period carbon dioxide elimination was 218.7 ml./min., whereas during meditation the mean was 186.8, a significant change (p < .005). Carbon dioxide elimination in the post-meditation period was near its pre-meditation level of 217.9 ml./min. (See Figure 5.17.) This simultaneous decrease in oxygen consumption and carbon dioxide elimination during meditation kept the so-called "respiratory quotient," which is simply the ratio of carbon dioxide elimination to oxygen consumption, at a relatively constant value of about .86 in the studies by Wallace. Dhanaraj [38] reported a relative constancy of respiratory quotient before and after meditation.

The partial pressures of carbon dioxide and oxygen in blood samples from the brachial artery were found by Wallace [39] to remain approximately constant during pre-meditation, meditative and post-meditation periods. (See Figure 5.20.) Wallace states, "After 6-7 hours of sleep and during high-voltage, slow-wave activity, O_2 consumption usually decreases about 15%." He adds that during sleep the partial pressure of carbon dioxide usually increases significantly, in contrast to its insignificant decrease during meditation. The constancy of arterial carbon dioxide pressure when combined with a slightly decreased base excess (also reported by Wallace; see Figure 5.21) indicates a "mild condition of metabolic acidosis" during meditation.

Hirai [40] found no noticeable increase in oxygen concentration in the blood of meditating Zen priests.

E. Endocrine and Nervous System Responses to Meditation

R. Jevning and his colleagues [41] determined concentrations of the hormones cortisol and prolactin in the blood of meditating subjects. Cortisol, as was mentioned in Chapter 4, is a hormone produced by the adrenal cortex gland. Prolactin is one of the many hormones produced by the anterior pituitary gland; it has a role in milk production in females and its level in the blood has been noted to increase with sleep onset. Seventeen subjects were studied by Jevning, 12 of whom had practiced meditation (Transcendental Meditation) for 3-5 years and 5 of whom had no meditative experience. Plasma cortisol and plasma prolactin levels were determined before, during and after a treatment period in which the long-term meditators practiced meditation and the controls rested with their eyes closed. The control group subjects then were taught meditation and, after 3 or 4 months of practice, were assayed for plasma prolactin before, during and after meditation. For both groups of meditators, average post-treatment values (see Figures 5.22 and 5.23) for plasma prolactin were greater than the treatment (meditation) period values; the differences were statistically significant ($p < .05$). For the long-term meditators, a small decrease in plasma cortisol level was seen during meditation; the difference between the pre-treatment and treatment (meditation) averages was statistically significant ($p < .05$). The average plasma cortisol values for the long-term meditators were less than for the control group which had not yet learned meditation. This finding suggests a decreased level of adrenal cortical activity as a result of long-term meditative practice; however, an experiment designed to control for group differences before meditation is learned would be needed to provide more conclusive support for this conjecture.

Udupa [42] reported that blood levels of acetylcholine and cholinesterase were significantly greater, in a group of subjects trained in meditation, after a meditation session than before.

Next, we will consider changes in the nervous system during meditation, limiting the discussion to changes in skin resistance. Wenger [43] found that the palmar conductance in both yoga students and older yoga practitioners decreased during the course of meditation. This finding indicates an increase in skin resistance during meditation. All conductance readings for the yoga students were higher during meditation than during a relaxation period. The decreases observed are consistent with muscular relaxation. (See Figure 4.12.)

Wallace (1970) [44] summarized that "skin resistance increased markedly at the onset of meditation, with some rhythmical fluctuations during meditation; it decreased to the resting value after meditation." For 15 subjects, the average increase in skin resistance during meditation was about 200% greater than the average skin resistance during rest prior to meditation. Large skin resistance increases occurred after only 10 minutes of meditation (see Figure 5.24). Wallace (1971) [45] stated that "in sleep skin resistance most commonly increases continuously, but the magnitude and rate of increase are generally less than that which occurred during meditation." For 36 subjects, an average increase in skin resistance of 258% over the pre-meditation period was found during meditation; this change was statistically significant ($p < .005$). Skin resistance was slightly higher during the post-meditation period. (See Figure 5.25.)

G. E. Schwartz [46] did not confirm the magnitude of skin resistance increases during meditation as reported by Wallace. In one experiment involving relatively short periods of meditation (Transcendental Meditation), skin resistance increases amounted to less than 20 kilohms and comparable increases in skin resistance were found in a control group who, instead of meditating, relaxed with eyes closed. In a second experiment,

Schwartz, in an attempt to replicate Wallace's experiments, again found only small increases in skin resistance. The reason for the apparent discrepancy between these two data sets of Wallace and Schwartz on skin resistance is not clear. Further work would be needed to clarify the nature of skin resistance changes during meditation. Schwartz suggests that the differences in the data sets may be due to the fact that Wallace, who personally knew many of the subjects in his experiment, provided an atmosphere more natural for the meditation of his subjects.

D. W. Orme-Johnson [47] compared subjects with experience in meditation (Transcendental Meditation) and control subjects without experience in meditation in terms of the number of spontaneous galvanic skin responses (GSR's), the rate of GSR habituation, and the number of multiple skin resistance responses to a stressful sound. Spontaneous GSR was defined as the sudden decrease in skin resistance of 100 ohms or more followed by resistance recovery, and such changes were counted only if they were independent of environmental noise or subject movement. Out of 13 measurements in 2 experimental groups, during meditation the number of spontaneous GSR's decreased (in comparison to a pre-treatment period) 10 times, increased 2 times and showed no change 1 time; for the controls during a period of rest with eyes closed the number of spontaneous GSR's decreased (in comparison to a pre-treatment period) 6 times in 15 measurements. The number of spontaneous GSR's was significantly less for meditative groups compared to controls, both while the groups rested with eyes open and while the meditators meditated and the controls rested with eyes closed. (See Figure 5.26.) Basal resistance of the two groups during rest with eyes closed did not differ significantly.

In studying the habituation of GSR response to a loud, unpleasant noise, Orme-Johnson found that for the first 11 presentations of the noise the habituation was similar in terms of latency and recovery time between the two groups and in terms of response amplitude.   However, the mean number of trials required to reach the criterion established for habituation was 11 for the meditators and 26.1 for the non-meditators. (See Figure 5.27.) Three of the non-meditators never achieved the habituation criterion before the session had to be ended, whereas all of the meditators did. The habituation experiments were not conducted during meditation but rather reflect the cumulative effects of meditation. The meditators made significantly fewer multiple skin resistance responses to the unpleasant noise than did the controls.

Hirai [48] found that a sound stimulus presented during a period of fast and slow alpha activity for a *zazen* meditator produced a galvanic skin response. Although GSR's ordinarily do not occur more than once every 10 seconds, more rapid succession of GSR's were observed occasionally for subjects during *zazen*.

·6·

EEG During Meditation

A. The EEG Rhythms

Turning now to examination of EEG research in meditation, we will first consider the changes in occurrence of the various frequency components of the EEG wave form; namely, the alpha, beta, theta ranges and certain other frequency components. For our purposes the range of frequencies will be roughly as follows:

beta and fast frequencies — 15 to 50 Hz.
alpha — 8 to 14 Hz.
theta — 4 to 7 Hz.
delta — 0 to 3 Hz.

When mention is made of a particular frequency, it will always be understood that the unit of the numbers referred to is the hertz (cycles per second). After discussion of the EEG frequency ranges that have been reported to occur during meditation, there will be considered the response of the EEG wave form in meditation to clicks and other stimuli.

A.1 Alpha Waves

The alpha rhythm is prominent in the EEG record from the occipital region when an individual closes his eyes; it remains prominent when a restful, non-problem solving mental state is retained.

As part of his work as consultant at the Menninger Foundation, Swami Rama demonstrated control over the production of various EEG patterns. First, he spent 5 fifteen-minute brainwave feedback sessions to learn "the relationship between the tones produced by activation in the various brain wave bands and the states of consciousness which he had learned" in his studies of yoga since early childhood. Then he produced various EEG patterns and described their subjective correlates. "He produced 70% alpha waves over a five-minute period of time by thinking of an empty blue sky 'with a small white cloud' sometimes coming by." He said after several alpha-producing sessions that "alpha isn't anything. It is literally nothing."[1]

Das found that his subjects when meditating showed acceleration of the alpha rhythm in the parietal, temporal and occipital regions by 1 to 3 Hz. above the normal frequency of 9 to 11 Hz. for these subjects in resting state.[2] This effect was accompanied by a decrease in the amplitude of the alpha waves. After certain EEG changes during the meditation period (see section A.4), all the subjects studied by Das showed a reappearance of the alpha rhythm after meditation, often with a decrease in frequency to 8 or even 7 Hz.

A. Kasamatsu[3] reported the EEG patterns among Zen masters and disciples in Japan. The recordings were made during the sitting with eyes partially open; the subjects were practicing *zazen*. For one Zen master, before the meditation, beta activity was apparent in all the EEG channels—frontal, central, parietal, occipital and parietal-occipital. Within 50 seconds or so after the Zen meditation was started, even though the eyes remained open there was an appearance of alpha waves at 11 to 12 Hz. with amplitudes ranging between 45 and 50 microvolts. After slightly more than 8 minutes of meditation, the amplitude of the alpha waves increased to include waves of 60 to 70 microvolts, the higher amplitudes occurring primarily in frontal and central regions. After 27 minutes, rhythmical waves of a lower frequency, 8 or even 7 Hz., appeared briefly. After certain further changes in the Zen master's EEG during *zazen* (see Section A.2), the alpha waves were seen to persist continuously for up to 2 minutes after the meditation; this record suggests an after-effect of the meditation.

A belt wave analyzer was employed by Hirai[4] to examine the kinds of alpha waves produced during *zazen* by 18 veteran Zen priests. In general, the priests emitted the same kinds of alpha waves. About 15 minutes after he began meditation, the parietal EEG of one priest showed large amplitude components of both slow (8-9 Hz.) and fast (10 Hz.) alpha waves, with only insiginificant quantities of other frequencies.

In his categorization of the EEG changes in Zen meditation, Kasamatsu posited 4 stages, the first of which is characterized by the appearance of alpha rhythm in spite of open eyes, the second of which is the increase in amplitude of persistent alpha and the third of which is the decrease of alpha frequency. The fourth stage will be described when we discuss the theta waves (see Section A.2 below). Of those Zen students who were evaluated by their instructors as "low" in their mental states, 5 reached during *zazen* no higher than the first EEG change just described, whereas 2 reached the second stage. Of those who were evaluated as "medium" in their mental state, 4 reached the first stage during *zazen*, 1 the second stage and the majority of 7 reached the third state as their highest stage reached during Zen meditation. (See Figure 6.1.)

Wallace (1971)[5] found that the intensity (mean square amplitude) of 8-9 Hz. slow alpha waves increased in the central and frontal regions during the middle part of meditation. The change in intensity of faster alpha waves at 10 to 11 Hz. was variable during meditation, while the intensity of the highest range of alpha of 12 to 14 Hz. either decreased or remained constant. In 3 subjects the EEG alpha was of low voltage during periods of reported drowsiness at the onset of meditation; however, as the meditation continued for these subjects, regular alpha activity replaced the low voltage alpha activity. Wallace (1970)[6] reported that in the EEG record of one subject during meditation the 9 Hz. alpha frequency showed the largest amplitude among alpha frequency components. At the beginning of meditation for this subject, there was an increase in the already rather high intensity of the 9 Hz. wave. During the middle of the subject's period of meditation, however, there was a considerable drop in the intensity of the 9 Hz. wave for a 2 to 5 minute interval, after which the intensity rapidly attained a value (about 1300 square microvolts) which was its maximum value during meditation. At the end of meditation the intensity of the 9 Hz. wave gradually decreased, even though the eyes remained closed.

F. M. Brown[7] found that 10 of 11 subjects during meditation showed the presence of frontal cortical alpha from 8 to 12 Hz. throughout most of a fifteen-minute period of meditation. In a control group of non-meditators, 3 of 11 subjects showed this pattern, although with less consistency than the meditating subjects, during a period in which they rested with their eyes closed. Frontal area alpha rhythm has been termed kappa rhythm activity; its occurrence is more rare than that of an occipital alpha rhythm.

Schwartz[8] found, in comparing a group of meditators with a matched group of controls, that upon entering the experiment the meditators showed more occipital alpha with eyes open than did the controls. After a brief eight-minute meditation, in which the controls rested with eyes closed, the meditators showed considerably less alpha with eyes open than did the controls. This finding was said by Schwartz to be consistent with subjective reports asserting the more striking appearance of visual stimuli after meditation. During meditation (or rest with eyes closed for the controls), each group showed marked increase in occipital alpha although the amount declined over the eight-minute experimental period, the decrease being somewhat greater for the control group.

The experimental procedure in the study of EEG in meditation by Banquet [9] consisted of an initial pre-meditation period of 5 minutes with eyes open and 5 minutes with eyes closed; a meditation period of about 30 minutes (or for the control group a period of 30 minutes relaxation with eyes closed); 3 minutes for a gradual coming out of relaxation or meditation; 5 minutes of mental concentration on a thought or image and then the opening of the eyes. There were 12 subjects in both the meditation and the control group. Those in the meditation group had practiced meditation from ¾ to 5 years, for an average of 2 years. EEG records were taken bilaterally from frontal, central, parietal and occipital regions, with linked ears for reference electrodes.

Banquet's control group showed during the test period either no stable alpha rhythm (4 subjects) or a constant alpha rhythm appearing in the posterior EEG channels (8 subjects). When coinciding with the decrease or disappearance of muscle artifacts in the EEG record, this type of EEG record was viewed as successful relaxation and was seen in 4 of the control subjects. The other 4 controls had alpha frequencies that were associated with EEG features characteristic of drowsiness and sleep, the alpha activity disappearing when sleep EEG patterns appeared.

Banquet found that most meditators, soon after beginning meditation, showed a predominance of the 10 Hz., 50 microvolts alpha waves that had been present in their resting EEG record. The amplitude increased sometimes to 70 microvolts. In 10 subjects the frequency decreased by 1 or 2 Hz., the decrease occurring first in the frontal EEG channel. These features characterized a first EEG stage of meditation delineated by Banquet, and this first stage was repeated at the end of meditation. At the end of the meditation period there was a great abundance of alpha waves, even more so than at the beginning of meditation.

In the second EEG stage of meditation as delineated by Banquet, if alpha waves appeared at all they appeared in short bursts lasting only a few seconds, generally spreading from occipital and parietal channels to frontal channels. There were periods of uniformity of frequency, amplitude and wave form of alpha in all the channels in both hemispheres. More unusual, according to Banquet, than the abundance of alpha in meditation in the beginning was "the ability of the meditators to maintain alpha activity after the end of meditation with eyes open as well as the diffusion of large amplitude alpha waves to anterior regions."

Anand,[10]   at the All-India Institute of Medical Sciences, studied the EEG obtained from 4 yogis before and during the practice of *samadhi*. The normal resting EEG of the yogis displayed a prominent alpha pattern. In *samadhi* the EEG of all subjects showed persistent alpha and, moreover, the alpha pattern showed a "well-marked increased amplitude modulation." The mononopolar EEG scalp records of one subject showed a predominant frequency of 11½ - 12 Hz. before and during meditation; in meditation, the EEG amplitude of this frequency, especially from occipital leads, increased to a maximum value of between 50 and 100 microvolts. One other subject showed occasional parietal hump activity.

Results of EEG experiments at Kaivalyadham on subjects practicing *dhyana* (meditation) were summarized by Swami Kuvalayananda[11] as follows:

When *Dhyana* is carried out successfully, it not only shows a reduction in the percentages of alpha-time, and a decrease in the amplitude of alpha waves . . . but the amplitude is lowered so much that it actually gives rise to an apparent 'flattening' of alpha. The alpha rhythm does not confine itself to occipital and parietal areas as usual, but is spread all over, and the flattening tendency too seems to be a general one.

The experiments in autonomic control with Swami Rama at the Menninger Foundation showed that during periods in which control over autonomically innervated activity, especially that of the heart, was being exercised, the EEG patterns consisted of low voltage activity.[12]

A.2 Theta Waves

Theta waves appear in the EEG ordinarily only in the transition between the waking state and the sleeping state, and have been associated with drowsiness.

Green [13] has found that training subjects through biofeedback procedures to produce theta waves has increased the occurrence of hypnogogic-like imagery which has been associated in other contexts with periods of high creativity.

In one five-minute experimental session at the Menninger Foundation, Swami Rama produced theta waves 75% of the time. This was done

by stilling the conscious mind and bringing forth the unconscious. [He further explained that the theta state was] very noisy. The things he had wanted to do but did not do, the things he should have done but did not do, and associated images and memories of people who wanted him to do things, came up in a rush and began shouting at him. It was a state that he generally kept turned off, he said, but it was also instructive and important to look in once in a while to see what was there.[14]

The fourth of the 4 stages of Zen meditation EEG patterns delineated by Kasamatsu [15] is the appearance of a rhythmical theta train. (See Section A.1 for a description of the first three stages.) In a Zen master it was found that 30 seconds after large amplitude slow frequency alpha waves had appeared during *zazen*, a rhythmical theta train with frequency of 6 to 7 Hz. and amplitude of 60 to 70 microvolts began to appear. "The appearance of the theta train becomes distinct throughout stable periods of large and slow alpha waves." Only Zen masters and 3 of 23 disciples studied showed this fourth stage during Zen meditation. These disciples were among those who had had the most experience in *zazen*, from 20 to 40 years, and they were also the ones evaluated by a Zen master as having a high mental state. The three other Zen disciples who had 20 to 40 years experience in *zazen* showed stage 3 EEG activity. Of those disciples studied who had from 5 to 20 years experience in *zazen*, one showed stage 1 EEG activity, one showed stage 2 activity and two showed stage 3 activity. Of those who had from 0 to 5 years experience in *zazen*, eight showed only stage 1 activity in Zen meditation, two showed stage 2 activity and three showed stage 3 activity. (See Figure 6.2.)

In 4 of the 15 subjects studied by Wallace (1970) [16] the alpha wave activity during meditation changed "to slower alpha wave frequency and in some cases stopped for 2-5 minutes and low-voltage theta waves predominated." In 5 of the 36 meditating subjects studied by Wallace (1971), [17] "the increased intensity of the 5-9 cycles/second activity was accompanied by occasional trains of 5-7 cycles/second waves (theta waves) in the frontal channel."

In the study of meditators by Banquet,[18] after the initial stage of the increased amplitude of alpha waves and the shift of alpha to lower frequencies (see Section A.1), a second EEG stage occurred in meditation.

> Within 5-20 minutes after the beginning of meditation short bursts of high voltage (up to 100 microvolts) theta waves at 5-7 c/sec occurred during 1 or 2 seconds, simultaneous in all channels, or first in the frontal region. Longer rhythmic theta trains (10 seconds to several minutes) at 60-80 microvolts usually followed. No further evolution in the meditation state happened in most subjects.

The theta frequency tended to appear first in frontal channels and then diffuse posteriorly. As with other EEG frequency ranges observed by Banquet, there were in all channels periods of uniformity of amplitude, frequency and wave form in the theta range. Theta waves sometimes persisted even into the eyes-open part of the post-meditation period.

A.3 Delta Waves

Delta waves are usually associated with deep sleep.

In a session at the Menninger Foundation, Swami Rama consciously produced delta waves during a twenty-five-minute period of what he termed "yogic sleep." During this period he was lying down with his eyes closed, snoring gently. Although his EEG and his observed activity were characteristic of deep sleep, Swami Rama continued to be conscious of occurrences in the experimental room. For example, one of the experimenters, without having previously mentioned that this would be done, every 5 minutes made a statement in a low voice in the experimental room. After the session, Swami Rama reported verbatim all these statements (except the fourth statement, which he paraphrased); also, he reported certain other environmental sounds that had occurred during this period. One of the experimenters wrote, "I was very much impressed because in listening from the control room, I had heard the sentences, but could not remember them all, and I was supposed to have been awake."

This paradoxical mixture of the waking state characteristic of environmental awareness with the sleep state characteristic of EEG delta waves remains to be fully explored and understood by scientists. Swami Rama explained [19] that in producing this delta state he had "told his mind to be quiet, to not respond to anything but to record everything, to remain in a deep state of tranquility until he activated it." He asserted that this yogic sleep was very beneficial, since " most people . . . let their brains go to sleep while their minds were still busy worrying over various matters, with the result that they woke up tired."

Next, we will consider delta waves as they have been reported to occur during meditation.

Wallace (1971) [20] reported that the intensity of delta wave components of frequency of 2-4 Hz. either decreased from its pre-meditation level or did not change during meditation. Three subjects who reported feeling drowsy at the beginning of meditation showed a decrease in alpha activity and showed a prominence of 2-7 Hz. EEG activity among low-voltage waves of mixed frequencies. Wallace (1970) [21] reported there were no delta waves or sleep spindles in EEG records of his subjects during meditation.

In 4 of the control subjects studied by Banquet [22] low-voltage delta activity occurred in conjunction with alpha activity and slow theta activity during the eyes-closed period. The EEG voltages during this time were relatively low, the frequencies were mixed, and drowsiness was reported by the control subjects. Two control subjects showed the high voltage delta wave characteristic of sleep and the simultaneous disappearance of alpha frequencies. There could occur during meditation "short bursts of large amplitude delta waves identical to those of sleep stage 4."

R. R. Pagano and colleagues [23] investigated the amount of time spent in sleep during meditation (Transcendental Meditation) and during a nap. He used as subjects five males, age 20 to 30 years, who had at least 2.5 years experience in the practice of Transcendental Meditation. EEG data from frontal, central and occipital leads were analyzed for each subject in 8 sessions, 4 in which the subject was asked to meditate in his usual way and 4 in which the subject was asked to nap lying on a bed for the same period. If he had meditated, at the end of the session the subject reported the depth of his meditation, and in all cases the subject reported whether he had slept or become drowsy during the session.

There was no significant correlation between the reported

depth of meditation (rated on a scale of 1 to 7) and the amount of time the subject slept. An analysis of variance of the amount of time spent by subjects in sleep stages 2, 3, or 4 showed no significant difference ($p < .1$) between the meditative sessions and the nap sessions. In one subject there were fewer EEG sleep patterns in meditation sessions than in nap sessions (t-test, $p < .01$); similar analyses for other subjects showed no significant differences between the meditative and nap sessions with respect to amount of time asleep. When EEG records of the meditation sessions were assessed for the amount of time in waking, stage 1 sleep (drowsiness) and stages 2, 3, 4 sleep (definitional sleep), it was found that 39% of the time subjects were awake, 19% of the time subjects were in stage 1 sleep, 23% of the time subjects were in stage 2 sleep and 17% of the time subjects were in stages 3 or 4 of sleep. Thus, 40% of the time during meditative sessions subjects were asleep (i.e., their EEG showed stages 2, 3 or 4 sleep patterns). Subjects reported (a) having slept in 12 of 13 meditation sessions where stage 2, 3 or 4 sleep occurred and (b) having felt drowsy in 18 of 19 sessions where more than 30 seconds of stage 1 sleep occurred. No rapid eye movements were noted in either the meditative or nap sessions.

A.4 Beta Waves

Beta waves in the EEG normally are associated with a subject's active attention to the outside world or to the solution of particular problems. If a person is awake with eyes open and is alert to his surroundings, normally the beta rhythm will be prominent in his EEG record.

In 4 of the meditating subjects studied by Banquet, a third stage, subsequent to the appearance of theta frequencies in the EEG, occurred and was accompanied by the push-button signal codes for deep meditation or transcendence. (See A.1 and A.2 for Banquet's first two stages.)

It was characterized by a pattern of generalized fast frequencies
with a dominant beta rhythm around 20 c/sec. Intermittent
spindle-like bursts alternated first with alpha or theta rhythms.
They showed a tendency to become continuous on a persistent
background of slower activity. This amplitude-modulated activity reached a surprisingly high voltage (30-60 microvolts). It
predominated in the anterior channels but was present and sometimes simultaneous in all of them.[24]

Spectral analysis indicated that in a period of transcendence, the
fast frequency had two components, one high voltage component
at 20 Hz. and another smaller voltage component at 40 Hz. The
20 Hz. beta rhythm was very stable in its frequency. In one case,
high voltage 20 Hz. beta activity occurred at the same time as
high voltage delta-theta activity. In one subject signalling the
transcendence stage, the amplitude-modulated beta activity was
apparent in all the EEG channels.

Beta frequencies, like theta frequencies, usually appeared
first in frontal channels and spread to posterior channels. Sometimes beta dominant activity occurred first in the left hemisphere,
from frontal to occipital channels, and then spread to the right
hemisphere.

Das [25] found beta activity during the practice of meditation
by his subjects. After the appearance of alpha waves of high frequency and lower amplitude, higher amplitude components at 15,
20 or 30 Hz. appeared in the EEG. Subsequently, a beta rhythm
from 16 to 20 Hz. appeared in the rolandic region, or there was an
increase in amplitude of such a rhythm if it had already appeared.
For some subjects, EEG activity generalized on both cerebral
hemispheres occurred at 20, 30 and sometimes even 40 Hz. The
amplitude of these fast EEG rhythms could reach a magnitude of
30 or even, in the case of a very deep meditation that reportedly
ended in *samadhi*, 50 microvolts. Immediately after the deepest
stage of meditation in one subject, occipital and temporal EEG
patterns at 18 Hz. occurred along with trains of generalized alpha
waves at 9 Hz. An hour after meditation, there remained for this

subject occipital rhythms at 9 Hz. and rolandic rhythms at 18 Hz. Das remarked that the stage considered as "ecstasy" was remarkable for the very high amplitude, rapid frequency waves present in all channels—frontal, central and occipital from both left and right hemispheres.

A.5 Other Aspects of EEG Rhythms

Norman Don [26] analyzed the EEG of a subject during an experience of an altered high state of consciousness. The EEG was characterized by simultaneous significant transient increases in amplitude of the predominant alpha, theta and delta frequencies. Don found this same pattern to be descriptive of the felt insight experiences with which his investigation was primarily concerned. The simultaneous appearance of high and low frequencies in deep meditative states, as reported by Banquet, is consistent with the pattern found by Don. Banquet reported that in the transitions among the 3 stages of EEG activity in meditation, "Two frequencies could appear simultaneously . . . : alpha and theta or slow and fast frequencies. If meditation lasted longer than the average 30 minutes several cycles took place."[27]

Green [28] remarked that when Swami Rama voluntarily produced high percentages of a given EEG frequency range, other frequency ranges did not cease. When Swami Rama produced alpha, the beta rhythm remained. When he produced theta, both alpha and beta rhythms remained, each about 50% of the time. When he produced delta, all 3 other types continued to remain in the EEG record.

Banquet [29] noted the tendency during meditation towards synchrony of the EEG pattern recorded from the various scalp leads. He stated that topographical changes in the EEG rhythm were of 2 types during meditation: first, "a constant tendency to synchronization of the anterior and posterior derivations," and second, "a transient asymmetry between right and left hemispheres . . . in the shifting phase from low to fast frequencies, with beta dominant activity appearing first in the left hemisphere."

B. EEG Responses to Stimuli

Some further insight into the EEG patterns in meditation may be obtained by examining the effect on EEG patterns of various stimuli presented during meditation.

Kasamatsu [30] reported that when click stimuli were repeated 20 times at 15-second intervals during periods of long persisting alpha in the EEG of a meditating Zen master, the alpha was repeatedly blocked; that is, the alpha changed to faster waves for 2 to 3 seconds. For resting control subjects alpha blocking occurred in response to the first few clicks, but the duration of the alpha blocking time was greatly decreased after many clicks were presented. In Zen masters the alpha blocking time during *zazen* remained fairly constant, with some random variations in length. This non-habituation of alpha blocking time in response to click stimuli during *zazen* is consistent with the description by one Zen master of the state of mind, cultivated in *zazen*, of "noticing every person one sees on the street but not looking back with emotional curiosity." The EEG response to a click stimulus in a certain Zen master when rhythmical theta trains predominated was a temporary blocking of the rhythmical theta train, which spontaneously reappeared several seconds afterwards. This shift from theta to beta is distinct from the transition from theta to alpha when drowsiness-related theta waves in the EEG are interrupted by a click. Kasamatsu characterized the state of mind during *zazen* as "relaxed awakening with steady responsiveness."

Whereas there is no habituation of blocking alpha EEG patterns by click stimuli in Zen meditation, there is, according to some investigators, no EEG change at all in response to click stimuli or other environmental stimuli during yoga meditation. Das [31] reported that during deep meditation, the EEG pattern of high amplitude beta waves was not changed by the appearance of auditory, visual, tactile or olfactory stimuli in the immediate physical environment of the subject. It was not reported whether such a subject mentioned afterwards that he was aware that such stimuli had been present.

Two of the 4 yogis whose EEG during *samadhi* was obtained by researchers [32] at the All-India Medical Institute were tested for reactivity to external stimuli during *samadhi*. The stimuli were photic (a strong light), auditory (a loud, banging noise), thermal (a touch with a hot glass tube) and vibratory (tuning fork). The presentation of these stimuli during *samadhi* evoked no changes in the EEG pattern. When questioned afterwards, the yogis did not report that they were aware of the presentation of these stimuli.

Swami Kuvalayananda [33] reported that even such painful stimuli as pin-pricks did not affect the generalized pattern of low-voltage EEG activity which he observed during *dhyana* (meditation).

The subject studied by Gharote [34] exhibited behavior whose description was similar. "He became quite unconscious to the environment and was not affected by such stimuli as shrill noise, touch, sharp prick, etc."

Banquet [35] reported that in the first stage of meditation (Transcendental Meditation), during the alpha periods there was usually no alpha blocking in response to flash or click stimuli. Nor did such stimuli change the EEG pattern of mixed slow and fast frequencies characteristic of deep meditation. The EEG pattern associated with deep meditation was not altered by mental activity or activity of the skeletal musculature involved in (a) use of the push-button signal to indicate mental activity or (b) memorization of and response to questions asked during the meditation period.

Certain reported features of response to stimuli in those practicing Transcendental Meditation, though inconsistent with findings on yoga, do seem consistent with the findings on *zazen*. Wallace (1970) [36] reported that "in almost all subjects, alpha blocking caused by reported sound or light stimuli showed no habituation." Banquet[37] reported that "rhythmic theta trains . . . were blocked by click stimuli but reappeared simultaneously within a few seconds . . . therefore, the rhythmic theta train of meditation has a reactivity similar to the waking alpha rhythm."

Appendices

Appendix A

References

INTRODUCTION
1. Swami Rama, *Lectures on Yoga.* Glenview, Illinois: Himalayan Institute, 1975.
2. Swami Kuvalayananda, *Popular Yoga Asanas.* Rutland, Vermont: Charles E. Tuttle Company, 1971.

CHAPTER 1
1. P. V. Karambelkar, M. V. Bhole, and M. L. Gharote, "Muscle Activity in Some Asanas," *Yoga-Mimamsa*, 12 (1): 1–13, July, 1969.
2. K. S. Gopal, V. Anatharaman, S. D. Nishith, and O. P. Bhatnagar, "The Effect of Yogasanas on Muscular Tone and Cardio-Respiratory Adjustments," *Yoga Life*, 6 (5): 3–11, May, 1975.
3. Swami Kuvalayananda, "X-Ray Experiments on Nauli," *Yoga-Mimamsa*, 1 (3): 168-185, 1925.
4. V. H. Dhanaraj, "The Effects of Yoga and the 5 BX Fitness Plan on Selected Physiological Parameters," Ph.D. dissertation, University of Alberta, 1974.
5. R. Moses, "Effect of Yoga on Flexibility and Respiratory Measures of Vital Capacity and Breath Holding Time," D. Ed. dissertation, University of Oregon, 1972.

6. M. L. Gharote, "Effect of Yogic Training on Physical Fitness," *Yoga-Mimamsa*, 15 (4): 31-35, 1973.

7. Swami Kuvalayananda, "X-Ray experiments on Uddiyana," *Yoga-Mimamsa*, 1(4): 250-254, 1925.

8. Swami Kuvalayananda, "Madhavadasa Vacuum," *Yoga-Mimamsa,* 1(2): 96-100, 1925.

9. M. V. Bhole, "Review of the Experimental Work Done on Uddiyana and Nauli in the Kaivalyadhama Laboratory," *Yoga-Mimamsa*, 15(1): 1-10, 1973.

10. M. A. Wenger and B. K. Bagchi, "Studies of Autonomic Functions in Practitioners of Yoga in India," *Behavioral Science*, 6: 312-323, 1961.

11. M. V. Bhole and P. V. Karambelkar, "Water Suction in Internal Cavities during Uddiyana and Nauli," *Yoga-Mimamsa,* 13(4): 26-32, 1971.

12. Swami Kuvalayananda, "Pressure Changes in Pranayama," *Yoga-Mimamsa,* 4(1): 47-61, 1930.

13. Swami Kuvalayananda, "Seven X-Ray Experiments Summed Up," *Yoga-Mimamsa,* 1(3): 190-191, 1925.

14. Swami Kuvalayananda and P. V. Karambelkar, "Kymographic and X-Ray Studies of Pressure Changes in Agnisara," *Yoga-Mimamsa,* 7(3): 157-167.

15. M. V. Bhole and P. V. Karambelkar, "Intra-gastric Pressure Changes in Asanas," *Yoga-Mimamsa,* 13(4): 67-73, 1971.

16. H. V. G. Rao, N. Krishnaswamy, R. L. Narasimhaiya, J. Hoenig, and M. V. Govindaswamy, "Some Experiments on a 'Yogi' in Controlled States," *Journal of the All-India Institute of Mental Health*, 1: 99-106, 1958.

17. Rudolph M. Ballentine, Jr., M.D. and Robert Gibbons, Unpublished manuscript, Forest Hospital and Himalayan Institute.

CHAPTER 2

1. S. K. Ganguly and M. L. Gharote, "Cardio-vascular Efficiency Before and After Yogic Training," Unpublished manuscript.

2. S. Rao, "Cardiovascular Responses to Head-Stand Posture," *Journal of Applied Physiology*, 18(5): 987-990, 1963.

3. K. S. Gopal, V. Anatharaman, S. D. Nishith, and O. P. Bhatnagar, "The Effect of Yogasanas on Muscular Tone and Cardio-Respiratory Adjustments," *Yoga Life*, 6(5): 3-11, May, 1975.

4. K. S. Gopal, V. Anantharaman, S. Balachander and S. D. Nishith, "The Cardiorespiratory Adjustments in 'Pranayama,' With and Without 'Bandhas,' in 'Vajrasana,' " *Indian Journal of Medical Science*, 27 (9): 686-672, September, 1973.

5. M. A. Wenger and B. K. Bagchi, "Studies of Autonomic Functions in Practitioners of Yoga in India," *Behavioral Science*, 6: 312-323, 1961.

6. E. E. Green, D. W. Ferguson, A. M. Green and E. D. Walters, *Preliminary Report on Voluntary Controls Project: Swami Rama*. Topeka, Kansas: The Menninger Foundation, 1970.

7. V. H. Dhanaraj, "The Effects of Yoga and the 5BX Fitness Plan on Selected Physiological Parameters," Ph.D. dissertation, University of Alberta, 1974.

8. Gopal, *et al.*, "The Effect of Yogasanas on Muscular Tone and Cardio-Respiratory Adjustments."

9. K. N. Udupa, R. H. Singh and R. M. Settiwar, "Studies on Physiological, Endocrine and Metabolic Response to the Practice of Yoga in Young Normal Volunteers," *Journal of Research in Indian Medicine*. 6 (3): 345-353, 1971.

10. K. N. Udupa, R. H. Singh, R. M. Settiwar and M. B. Singh, "Physiological and Biochemical Changes

Following the Practice of Some Yogic and Non-Yogic Exercises," *Journal of Research in Indian Medicine*. 10 (2): 91-93, 1975.

11.   Udupa, *op. cit.*

12.   Udupa, *et al.*, "Physiological and Biochemical Changes."

13.   See both preceeding references by Gopal, *et al.*

14.   *Ibid.*

15.   Dhanaraj, *op. cit.*

16.   Rao, *op. cit.*

17.   Dhanaraj, *op. cit.*

18.   Wenger, *op. cit.*

19.   Dhanaraj, *op. cit.*

20.   K. S. Gopal, O. P. Bhatnagar, N. Subramanian and S. D. Nishith, "Effect of Yogasanas and Pranayamas on Blood Pressure, Pulse Rate and Some Respiratory Functions," *Indian Journal of Physiology and Pharmacy*. 17 (3): 273-276, July, 1973.

21.   Dhanaraj, op. cit.

22.   *Ibid.*

23.   H. V. G. Rao, N. Krishnaswamy, R. L. Narasimhaiya, J. Hoenig, and M. V. Govindaswamy, "Some Experiments on a 'Yogi' in Controlled States," *Journal of the All-India Institute of Mental Health*. 1: 99-106, 1958.

24.   Rudolph M. Ballentine, Jr., M.D. and Robert Gibbons, Unpublished manuscript, Forest Hospital and Himalayan Institute.

25.   B. K. Anand, G. S. Chhina, and B. Singh, "Studies on Shri Ramanand Yogi During His Stay in an Air-Tight Box," *Indian Journal of Medical Research*, 49 (1): 82-89, January, 1961.

26.   P. V. Karambelkar, S. L. Vinekar and M. V. Bhole, "Studies on Human Subjects Staying in an Air-Tight Pit," *Indian Journal of Medical Research*, 56 (8): 1282-1288, 1968.

27.   C. Laubry and T. Brosse, "Data Gathered in India on a Yogi with Simultaneous Registration of the Pulse, Respiration and Electrocardiogram," *Presse Medicale*, 44: 1601-1604, 1936.

28.   M. A. Wenger, B. K. Bagchi and B. K. Anand, "Experiments in India on 'Voluntary' Control of the Heart and Pulse," *Circulation*, 24:   1319-1325, December 1961.

29.   M. V. Bhole and P. V. Karambelkar, "Heart Control and Yoga Practices," *Yoga-Mimamsa*, 13 (4): 53-65, 1971.

30.   Green, *et al., op. cit.*

31.   L. K. Kothari, A. Bordia and O. P. Gupta, "The Yogic Claim of Voluntary Control over the Heart Beat: an Unusual Demonstration," *American Heart Journal*, 86: 282-284, 1973.

32.   Rao, *op. cit.*

33.   (a) Swami Kuvalayananda, "Blood Pressure Experiments on Sarvangasana and Matsyasana," *Yoga-Mimamsa*, 2 (1): 12-38, 1926.
      (b) Swami Kuvalayananda, "Blood Pressure Experiments on Shirshasana, " *Yoga-Mimamsa*, 2 (1): 92-99, 1926.

34.   Wenger, *op. cit.*

35.   Karambelkar, *et al. op cit.*

36.   Gopal, Bhatnagar, Subramanian and Nishith, *op. cit.*

37.   Udupa, Singh, and Settiwar, *op. cit.*

38.   Udupa, Singh, Settiwar and Singh, *op. cit.*

39.   K. K. Datey, S. Deshmukh, C. Dalvi and S. L. Vinekar, "Shavasana: A Yogic Exercise in the Management of Hypertension," *Angiology*, 20: 325-333, 1969.

40.   C. H. Patel, "Yoga and Bio-Feedback in the Management of Hypertension," *Lancet*: 1053-1055, November 10, 1973.

41.   C. H. Patel, "12-Month Follow-up of Yoga and Bio-

feedback in Management of Hypertension," *Lancet*: 93-95, July 19, 1975.

43. Dhanaraj, *op. cit.*

44. M. V. Bhole and P. V. Karambelkar, "Effect of Yogic Treatment on Blood Picture in Asthma Patients," *Yoga-Mimamsa*, 14 (1 & 2): 1-6, April and July, 1971.

45. M. V. Bhole, "Treatment of Bronchial Asthma by Yogic Methods," *Yoga-Mimamsa*, 9 (3): 33-41, January, 1967.

46. Udupa, Singh, Settiwar and Singh, *op. cit.*

47. K. S. Gopal, A. Natarajan and S. Ramakrishnan, "Biochemical Studies in Foreign Volunteers Practicing Hatha Yoga," *Journal of Research in Indian Medicine*, 9 (3): 1-8, 1974.

CHAPTER 3

1. V. Pratap, "Diurnal Pattern of Nostril Breathing—An Exploratory Study," *Yoga-Mimamsa*, 14 (3 & 4): 1-17, October, 1971 and January, 1972.

2. M. V. Bhole and P. V. Karambelkar, "Significance of Nostrils in Breathing," *Yoga-Mimamsa*, 10 (4): 1-12, April, 1968.

3. S. Rao and A. Potdar, "Nasal Airflow with Body in Various Positions," *Journal of Applied Physiology*, 28 (2): 162-165, 1970.

4. K. N. Udupa, R. H. Singh and R. M. Settiwar, "Studies on Physiological, Endocrine and Metabolic Response to the Practice of Yoga in Young Normal Volunteers," *Journal of Research in Indian Medicine*, 6 (3): 345-353, 1971.

5. K. N. Udupa, R. H. Singh, R. M. Settiwar and M. B. Singh, "Physiological and Biochemical Changes Following the Practice of Some Yogic and Non-Yogic Exercises," *Journal of Research in Indian Medicine*, 10 (2): 91-93, 1975.

6. V. H. Dhanaraj, "The Effects of Yoga and the 5BX Fitness Plan on Selected Physiological Parameters," Ph.D. dissertation, University of Alberta, 1974.

7. K. S. Gopal, V. Anantharaman, S. Balachander and S. D. Nishith, "The Cardiorespiratory Adjustments in 'Pranayama,' With and Without 'Bandhas,' in 'Vajrasana,' " *Indian Journal of Medical Science*, 27 (9): 686-672, September, 1973.

8. K. S. Gopal, V. Anatharaman, S. D. Nishith, and O. P. Bhatnagar, "The Effect of Yogasanas on Muscular Tone and Cardio-Respiratory Adjustments," *Yoga Life*, 6 (5): 3-11, May, 1975.

9. M. A. Wenger and B. K. Bagchi, "Studies of Autonomic Functions in Practitioners of Yoga in India," *Behavioral Science*, 6: 312-323, 1961.

10. C. H. Patel, "Yoga and Bio-Feedback in the Management of Hypertension," *Lancet*: 1053-1055, November 10, 1973.

11. Dhanaraj, *op. cit.*

12. S. Rao, "Respiratory Responses to Headstand Posture," *Journal of Applied Physiology*, 24 (5): 697-699, 1968.

13. W. R. Miles, "Oxygen Consumption During Three Yoga-Type Breathing Patterns," *Journal of Applied Physiology*, 19 (1): 75-82, 1964.

14. S. Rao, "Oxygen Consumption During Yoga-Type Breathing at Altitudes of 520 m. and 3,800 m.," *Indian Journal of Medical Research*, 56 (5): 701-705, 1968.

15. P. V. Karambelkar, S. L. Vinekar and M. V. Bhole, "Studies on Human Subjects Staying in an Air-Tight Pit," *Indian Journal of Medical Research*, 56 (8): 1282-1288, 1968.

16. C. Laubry and T. Brosse, "Data Gathered in India on a Yogi with Simultaneous Registration of the Pulse, Respiration and Electrocardiogram," *Presse Medicale*, 44: 1601-1604, 1936.

17.   H. V. G. Rao, N. Krishnaswamy, R. L. Narasimhaiya, J. Hoenig and M. V. Govindaswamy, "Some Experiments on a 'Yogi' in Controlled States," *Journal of the All-India Institute of Mental Health*, 1: 99-106, 1958.

18.   Rudolph M. Ballentine, Jr., M.D. and Robert Gibbons, Unpublished Manuscript, Forest Hospital and Himalayan Institute.

19.   M. V. Bhole and P. V. Karambelkar, "Effect of Yoga Training on Vital Capacity and Breath-Holding Time—A Study," *Yoga-Mimamsa*, 14 (3 & 4): 19-26, 1971.

20.   K. S. Gopal, O. P. Bhatnagar, N. Subramanian and S. D. Nishith, "Effect of Yogasanas and Pranayamas on Blood Pressure, Pulse Rate and Some Respiratory Functions," *Indian Journal of Physiology and Pharmacy*. 17 (3): 273-276, July, 1973.

21.   Dhanaraj, *op. cit.*

22.   (a) Udupa, Singh and Settiwar, *op. cit.*
      (b) Udupa, Singh, Settiwar and Singh, *op. cit.*

23.   R. Moses, "Effect of Yoga on Flexibility and Respiratory Measures of Vital Capacity and Breath Holding Time," D. Ed. dissertation, University of Oregon, 1972.

24.   Gopal, Anantharaman, Balachander and Nishith, *op. cit.*

25.   Gopal, Anantharaman, Nishith and Bhatnagar, *op. cit.*

26.   Datey, *op. cit.*

27.   Udupa, Singh and Settiwar, *op. cit.*

28.   Dhanaraj, *op. cit.*

29.   K. S. Gopal and S. Lakshmanan, "Some Observations on Hatha Yoga: The Bandhas, an Anatomical Study," *Yoga Life*, 4 (1): 3-18, January, 1973.

30.   Rao, "Respiratory Responses to Headstand Posture," *op. cit.*

31.   Rao, "Oxygen Consumption during Yoga-Type Breathing," *op. cit.*

32.   Dhanaraj, *op. cit.*

33. Gopal, Bhatnagar, Subramanian and Nishith, *op. cit.*
34. Dhanaraj, *op. cit.*
35. Rao, "Respiratory Responses to Headstand Posture," *op. cit.*
36. Miles, *op. cit.*
37. Rao, "Oxygen Consumption during Yoga-Type Breathing," *op. cit.*
38. Udupa, Singh and Settiwar, *op. cit.*
39. Dhanaraj, *op. cit.*
40. Gopal, Bhatnagar, Subramanian and Nishith, *op. cit.*
41. Moses, *op. cit.*
42. M. V. Bhole, D. V. Karambelkar, and M. L. Gharote, "Effect of Yoga Practices on Vital Capacity," *Indian Journal of Chest Disease*, 12 (1 & 2): 32-35, 1970.
43. Udupa, Singh and Settiwar, *op. cit.*
44. Rao, "Respiratory Responses to Headstand Posture," *op. cit.*
45. *Ibid.*
46. Gopal, Bhatnagar, Subramanian and Nishith, *op. cit.*
47. Dhanaraj, *op. cit.*
48. S. C. B. Rangan, "An Experimental Study to Investigate the Effect of Sarvangasana and Halasana," M. P. E. Thesis, Lakshmibai College of Physical Education, Gwalior, India, 1969.
49. D. C. Salgar, V. S. Bisen, and M. J. Jinturkar, "Effect of Padmasana—A Yogic Exercise—on Muscular Efficiency," *Indian Journal of Medical Research*, 63 (6): 68-72, June, 1975.
50. Dhanaraj, *op. cit.*
51. Salgar, *op. cit.*
52. S. Rao, "Metabolic Cost of Head-stand Posture," *Journal of Applied Physiology*, 17 (1): 117-118, 1962.
53. Swami Kuvalayananda, "Blood Pressure Experiments on Sirsasana," *Yoga-Mimamsa*, 2 (2): 92-99, 1926.
54. Miles, *op. cit.*

55. Rao, "Oxygen Consumption during Yoga-Type Breathing," *op. cit.*

56. Swami Kuvalayananda and P. V. Karambelkar, "Studies in Alveolar Air during Kapalabhati," *Yoga-Mimamsa,* 7 (2): 87-94, 1957.

57. (a) Swami Kuvalayananda, "CO_2 Elimination in Pranayama," *Yoga-Mimamsa,* 4 (2): 95-120, 1930.
    (b) Swami Kuvalayananda, "O_2 Absorbtion and CO_2 elimination in Pranayama," *Yoga-Mimamsa,* 4 (4): 267-289, 1933.

58. H. V. G. Rao, *et. al., op. cit.*

59. Rudolph M. Ballentine, Jr., M.D. and Robert Gibbons, Unpublished Manuscript, Forest Hospital and Himalayan Institute.

60. Karambelkar, Vinekar and Bhole, *op. cit.*

61. Anand, Chhina and Singh, *op. cit.*

CHAPTER 4

1. V. H. Dhanaraj, "The Effects of Yoga and the 5BX Fitness Plan on Selected Physiological Parameters," Ph.D. dissertation, University of Alberta, 1974.

2. K. N. Udupa, R. H. Singh and R. M. Settiwar, "Studies on Physiological, Endocrine and Metabolic Response to the Practice of Yoga in Young Normal Volunteers," *Journal of Research in Indian Medicine,* 6 (3): 345-353, 1971.

3. K. N. Udupa, R. H. Singh, R. M. Settiwar and M. B. Singh, "Physiological and Biochemical Changes Following the Practice of Some Yogic and Non-Yogic Exercises," *Journal of Research in Indian Medicine,* 10 (2): 91-93, 1975.

4. *Ibid.*

5. P. V. Karambelkar, M. V. Bhole and M. L. Gharote, "Effect of Yogic Asanas on Uropepsin Excretion," *Indian Journal of Medical Research,* 57 (5): 944-947,

May, 1969.

6.   Udupa, Singh, Settiwar and Singh, *op. cit.*

7.   K. N. Udupa, R. H. Singh and R. A. Yadav, "Certain Studies on Psychological and Biochemical Responses to the Practice of Hatha Yoga in Young Normal Volunteers," *Indian Journal of Medical Research,* 61 (2): 237-244, 1973.

8.   M. L. Gharote, "A Psychophysiological Study of the Effects of Short-term Yogic Training on the Adolescent High School Boys," *Yoga-Mimamsa,* 14 (1 & 2): 92-99, 1971.

9.   M. A. Wenger and B. K. Bagchi, "Studies of Autonomic Functions in Practitioners of Yoga in India," *Behavioral Science,* 6: 312-323, 1961.

10.   V. Pratap, "Difference in Magnitude of Response in Yogic and Non-Yogic Conditions," *Yoga-Mimamsa,* 12 (2): 9-18, October, 1969.

11.   C. Laubry and T. Brosse, "Data Gathered in India on a Yogi with Simultaneous Registration of the Pulse, Respiration and Electrocardiogram," *Presse Medicale,* 44: 1601-1604, 1936.

12.   P. V. Karambelkar, S. L. Vinekar and M. V. Bhole, "Studies on Human Subjects Staying in an Air-Tight Pit," *Indian Journal of Medical Research* 56 (8): 1282-1288, 1968.

13.   H. V. G. Rao, N. Krishnaswamy, R. L. Narasimhaiya, J. Hoenig and M. V. Govindaswamy, "Some Experiments on a 'Yogi' in Controlled States," *Journal of the All-India Institute of Mental Health,* 1: 99-106, 1958.

14.   Rudolph M. Ballentine, Jr., M.D. and Robert Gibbons, Unpublished Manuscript, Forest Hospital and Himalayan Institute.

15.   T. Hirai, *Zen Meditation Therapy.* Tokyo: Japan Publications, 1975.

16. J. V. Hardt, *Relaxation During Breathing Feedback, Yogic Breathing, and Alpha Feedback.* San Francisco: Langley Porter Neuropsychiatric Institute.

17. B. Timmons, J. Salamy, J. Kamiya, and D. Girtan, "Abdominal-Thoracic Respiratory Movements and Levels of Arousal," *Psychon. Sci.*, 27 (3): 173-175, 1972.

CHAPTER 5

1. Swami Rama, *Lectures on Yoga.* Glenview, Illinois: Himalayan Institute, 1975.

2. N. N. Das and H. Gastant, "Variations de l'Activité Electrique du Cerveau, du Coeur et des Muscles Squelettiques au Cours de la Méditation et de l'Extase Yogique," *EEG*, Supplement 6: 211-219, 1955.

3. R. K. Wallace, "Physiological Effects of Transcendental Meditation," *Science*, 167: 1751-1754, March 27, 1970.

4. T. Hirai, *Zen Meditation Therapy.* Tokyo: Japan Publications, 1975.

5. Das and Gastaut, *op. cit.*

6. J. P. Banquet, "Spectral Analysis of the EEG in Meditation," *Electroencephalography and Clinical Neurophysiology*, 35: 143-151, 1973.

7. M. A. Wenger and B. K. Bagchi, "Studies of Autonomic Functions in Practitioners of Yoga in India," *Behavioral Science*, 6: 312-323, 1961.

8. H. Rieckert, "Plethysmographic Studies on Concentration and Meditation Exercises," *Arztliche Forschung*, 21: 61-65, 1967.

9. V. L. Levander, H. Benson, R. C. Wheeler and R. K. Wallace, "Increased Forearm Blood Flow during a Wakeful Hypometabolic State," *Federation Proc.*, 31 (2): 405, March-April, 1972.

10. R. K. Wallace, H. Benson and A. F. Wilson, "A Wakeful Hypometabolic Physiologic State," *Am. J. Physiology*, 221 (3): 795-799, 1971.

11. Wenger and Bagchi, *op. cit.*

12. Wallace, *et al., op. cit.*

13. H. Benson, B. A. Rosner, B. R. Marzetta and H. M. Klemchuk, "Decreased Blood-Pressure in Pharmacologically Treated Hypertensive Patients who Regularly Elicited the Relaxation Response," *Lancet:* 289-291, 1974.

14. Wallace, *op. cit.*

15. Wallace, *et al, op. cit.*

16. V. H. Dhanaraj, "The Effects of Yoga and the 5BX Fitness Plan on Selected Physiological Parameters," Ph.D. dissertation, University of Alberta, 1974.

17. Wenger and Bagchi, *op. cit.*

18. Das and Gastant, *op. cit.*

19. Hirai, *op. cit.*

20. Wallace, *et. al., op. cit.*

21. Hirai, *op. cit.*

22. *Ibid.*

23. Wenger and Bagchi, *op. cit.*

24. Dhanaraj, *op. cit.*

25. Wallace, *et al., op. cit.*

26. J. Allison, "Respiratory Changes during the Practice of the Technique of Transcendental Meditation," *Lancet,* 833-834, 1970.

27. Dhanaraj, *op. cit.*

28. Wallace, *et al., op. cit.*

29. Wallace, *op. cit.*

30. Wallace, et al., op. cit.

31. H. Benson, J. F. Beary and M. P. Carol, "The Relaxation Response," *Psychiatry,* 37: 37-46, 1974.

32. Dhanaraj, *op. cit.*

33. Wallace, *op. cit.*

34. Wallace, *et al., op. cit.*

35. Reported in Hirai, *op. cit.*

36. M. L. Gharote, "Energy Expenditure during Deep

37. Wallace, *et al., op. cit.*
38. Dhanaraj, *op. cit.*
39. Wallace, *et al., op. cit.*
40. Hirai, *op. cit.*
41. R. Jevning, A. Wilson, E. Vanderlaan and S. Levine, "Plasma Prolactin and Cortisol during Transcendental Meditation." In D. W. Orme-Johnson and J. T. Farrow, eds., *Scientific Research on the Transcendental Meditation Program, Collected Papers, Volume 1.* Special prepublication copy.
42. K. N. Udupa, R. H. Singh and R. M. Settiwar, "Studies on Physiological, Endocrine and Metabolic Response to the Practice of Yoga in Young Normal Volunteers," *Journal Research in Indian Medicine*, 6 (3): 345-353, 1971.
43. Wenger and Bagchi, *op. cit.*
44. Wallace, *op. cit.*
45. Wallace, *et al., op. cit.*
46. G. E. Schwartz, "Pros and Cons of Meditation," (paper presented at the American Psychological Association Convention, Montreal, August, 1973).
47. D. W. Orme-Johnson, "Autonomic Stability and Transcental Meditation," *Psychosomatic Medicine*, 35: 341-349, 1973.
48. Hirai, *op. cit.*

CHAPTER 6

1. E. E. Green, A. M. Green, E. D. Walters, *Biofeedback for Mind-Body Self-Regulation: Healing and Creativity.* Topeka, Kansas: The Menninger Foundation, 1971.
2. Swami Rama, *Lectures on Yoga.* Glenview, Illinois: Himalayan Institute, 1975.
3. A. Kasamatsu and R. Hirai, "An Electroencephalographic Study on the Zen Meditation (Zazen)," in *Altered States of Consciousness*, ed. C. T. Tart, Garden

City, New York: Doubleday, 1972, pp. 501-514.

4. H. V. G. Rao, N. Krishnaswamy, R. L. Narasimhaiya, J. Hoenig and M. V. Govindaswamy, "Some Experiments on a 'Yogi' in Controlled States," *Journal of the All-India Institute of Mental Health,* 1: 99-106, 1958.

5. J. P. Banquet, "Spectral Analysis of the EEG in Meditation," *Electroencephalography and Clinical Neurophysiology,* 35: 143-151, 1973.

6. Wenger and Bagchi, *op. cit.*

7. F. M. Brown, W. S. Stewart and J. T. Blodgett, "EEG Kappa Rhythms during Transcendental Meditation and Possible Threshold Changes Following," (paper presented to the Kentucky Academy of Science, Richmond, November 13, 1971).

8. K. N. Udupa, R. H. Singh and R. M. Settiwar, "Studies on Physiological, Endocrine and Metabolic Response to the Practice of Yoga in Young Normal Volunteers," *Journal of Research in Indian Medicine,* 6 (3): 345-353, 1971.

9. N. N. Das and H. Gastant, "Variations de l'Activité Electrique du Cerveau, du Coeur et des Muscles Squelettiques au Cours de la Méditation et de l'Extase Yogique," *EEG,* Supplement 6: 211-219, 1955.

10. B. K. Anand, G. S. Chhina and Baldev Singh, "Some Aspects of Electroencephalographic Studies in Yogis," *EEG and Clinical Neurophysiology,* 13: 452-456, 1961.

11. Swami Kuvalayananda and S. L. Vinekar, *Yogic Therapy: Its Basic Principles and Methods.* New Delhi: Ministry of Health, Government of India, 1971.

12. E. E. Green, D. W. Ferguson, A. M. Green, and E. D. Walters, *Preliminary Report on Voluntary Controls Project: Swami Rama.* Topeka, Kansas: The Menninger Foundation, 1970.

13. A. M. Green, E. E. Green, and E. D. Walters, *Brainwave Training, Imagery, Creativity and Integrative Experiences.* Topeka, Kansas: The Menninger Foundation, 1973.

14. Green, *et al., Biofeedback for Mind-Body Self-Regulation, op. cit.*

15. Kasamatsu and Hirai, *op. cit.*

16. Wallace, *op. cit.*

17. Wallace, *et al., op. cit.*

18. Banquet, *op. cit.*

19. Green, *et al., Biofeedback for Mind-Body Self-Regulation, op. cit.*

20. Wallace, *et al., op. cit.*

21. Wallace, *op. cit.*

22. Banquet, *op. cit.*

23. R. R. Pagano, R. M. Rose, R. M. Stivers, and S. Warrenburg, "Sleep during Transcendental Meditation," *Science* 191: 308-310, 23 January, 1976.

24. Banquet, *op. cit.*

25. Das and Gastaut, *op. cit.*

26. N. S. Don, *Cortical Activity Change during a Psychotherapeutic Procedure: A Model for Changes of States of Awareness.* Chicago: Pritzker School of Medicine, University of Chicago, 1974.

27. Banquet, *op. cit.*

28. Green, *et al., Biofeedback for Mind-Body Self-Regulation, op. cit.*

29. Banquet, *op. cit.*

30. Kasamatsu and Hirai, *op. cit.*

31. Das and Gastaut, *op. cit.*

32. Anand, *et al., op. cit.*

33. Kuvalayananda and Vinekar, *op. cit.*

34. M. L. Gharote, "Energy Expenditure during Deep Meditative State," *Yoga-Mimamsa*, 14 (1 & 2): 57-62, 1971.

35.   Banquet, *op. cit.*
36.   Wallace, *op. cit.*
37.   Banquet, *op. cit.*

Appendix B

Figures

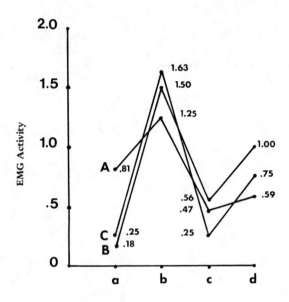

Figure 1.1

Change (Before Minus After) in EMG
Activity. (Karambelkar, *et al.*)[1]

A = Half-Spinal Twist (Left)
B = Posterior Stretching Posture
C = Half-Spinal Twist (Right)

a = Back
b = Buttock
c = Thigh
d = Calf

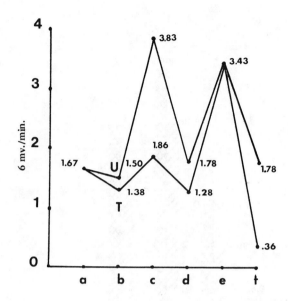

Figure 1.2

EMG (Non-integrated)
in Various Asanas.
(Gopal, *et al.*)[2]

T = Trained Subjects
U = Untrained Subjects

a = Inverted Action
b = Shoulder stand
c = Headstand
d = Bridge Posture
e = Half-Spinal Twist
f = Symbol of Yoga

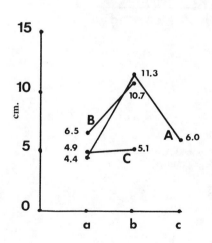

Figure 1.3

Flexibility (Wells Sit-and-Reach Test).
(Dhanaraj)[4]

A = Yoga Group
B = 5BX Group
C = Control Group

a = Pre-training
b = Post-training (6 weeks)
c = Post-detraining (6 weeks, yoga
    group only)

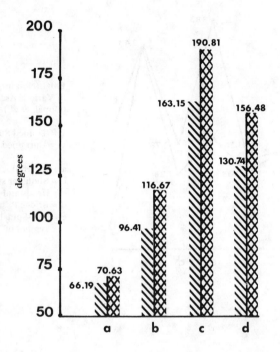

Figure 1.4

Flexibility Before and After
10 Weeks of Yoga. (Moses)[5]

///// = Before
XXXX = After

a = Ankle
b = Hip
c = Hip and Trunk
d = Neck

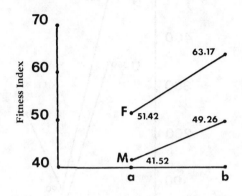

Figure 1.5

Physical Fitness Index Before
and After 3 Weeks of Yoga.
(Gharote)[6]

F = Females, based on four
    tests
M = Males, based on eight
    tests

a = Before
b = After

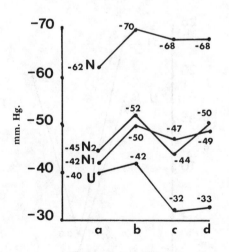

Figure 1.6

Internal Pressures During
Abdominal Lock and Nauli.
(Bhole)[9]

N   = Nauli (Middle)
N1 = Nauli (Right Side)
N2 = Nauli (Left Side)
U   = Abdominal Lock

a = Esophagus
b = Stomach
c = Colon
d = Bladder

Figure 1.7

Water Suction Volume. (Bhole
and Karambelkar)[11]

N = Nauli
U = Abdominal Lock

a = Stomach
b = Bladder
c = Colon

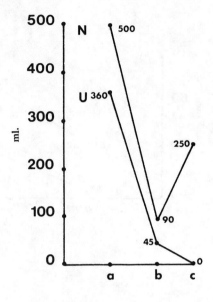

Figure 1.8

Water Suction Rate. (Bhole and
Karambelkar)[11]

N = Nauli
U = Abdominal Lock

a = Stomach
b = Bladder
c = Colon

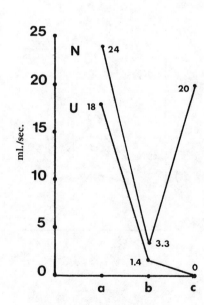

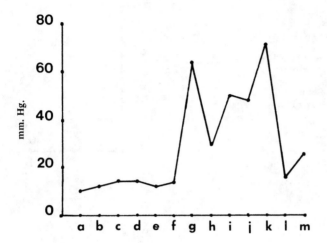

Figure 1.9

Intragastric Pressure During Asanas.
(Bhole and Karambelkar)[14]

a = Headstand
b = Shoulder stand
c = Fish Posture
d = Plow Posture
e = Half-Locust Pose (Right)
f = Half-Locust Post (Left)
g = Locust Posture
h = Cobra Posture
i = Bow Posture
j = Boat Posture
k = Peacock Posture
l = Half-Spinal Twist (Right)
m = Half-Spinal Twist (Left)

Figure 2.1

Harvard Step Test. (Ganguly
and Gharote)[1]

a = Before
b = After 9 mos. of Yoga

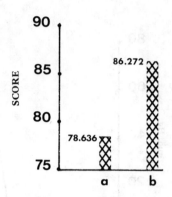

Figure 2.2

Harvard Step Test. (Ganguly
and Gharote)[1]

A = Initial Hi-Ave. Subjects
B = Initial Good Subjects

a = Final Hi-Ave. (65-79)
b = Final Good (80-89)
c = Final Excellent (90-)

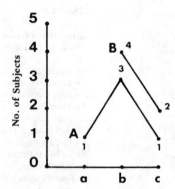

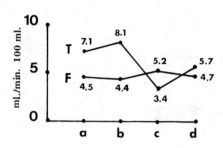

Figure 2.3

Blood Flow with Body in Various Positions. (Rao)[2]

F = Finger Blood Flow
T = Toe Blood Flow

a = Horizontal Supine Position
b = Erect Standing Position
c = Headstand Position
d = Horizontal Supine Position

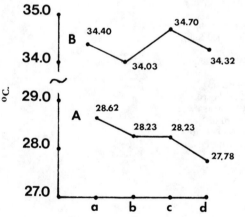

Figure 2.4

Skin Temperature
with Body in Various
Positions. (Rao)[2]

A = Dorsum Foot Temperature
B = Forehead Temperature

a = Horizontal Supine Position
b = Erect Standing Position
c = Headstand Position
d = Horizontal Supine Position

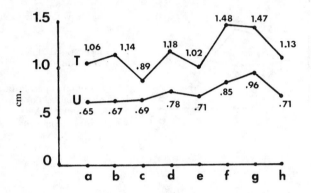

Figure 2.5

Peripheral Blood Flow
(Amplitude of Electrical Trans-
duction). (Gopal, *et al.*)[3]

T = Trained Subjects
U = Untrained Subjects

a = Inverted Action
b = Shoulder stand
c = Headstand
d = Bridge Posture
e = Half-Spinal Twist
f = Symbol of Yoga
g = Corpse Posture
h = Adamant Posture

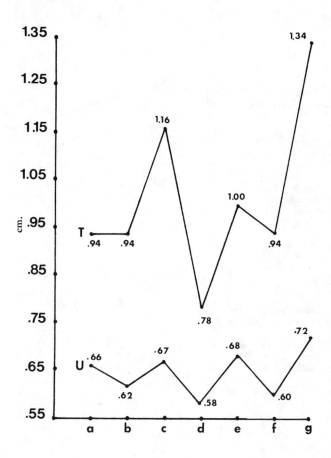

Figure 2.6

Peripheral Blood Flow in Various Breathing Patterns. (Gopal, *et al.*)[4]

T = Trained Subjects
U = Untrained Subjects

a = Normal Rhythmic Breathing; b = Rhythmic Inspiration (inhale for 7 counts, retain for 14 counts); c = Rhythmic Expiration (Exhale for 7 counts, retain for 14 counts); d = Deep Inspiration with Locks; e = Deep Expiration with Locks; f = Deep Inspiration with Locks; g = Deep Expiration without Locks.

Figure 2.7

Finger Temperature During Breathing
Practices. (Wenger and Bagchi)[5]

A = Ujjayi
B = Bhastrika (Bellows)
C = Hyperventilation after
     Bhastrika

a = Pre-Exercise Period
b = Exercise Period
c = Post-Exercise Period

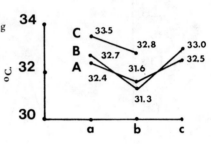

Figure 2.8

Finger Temperature During Breathing
Practices. (Wenger and Bagchi)[5]

A = Kapalabhati (Skull-shining)
B = Hyperventilation after
     Kapalabhati

a = Pre-Exercise Period
b = Exercise Period

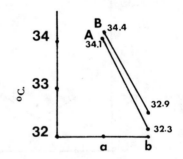

Figure 2.9

Finger Pulse Volume During
Breathing Practices. (Wenger
and Bagchi)[5]

A = Ujjayi
B = Bhastrika (Bellows)
C = Hyperventilation after
     Bhastrika

a = Pre-Exercise Period
b = Exercise Period
c = Post-Exercise Period

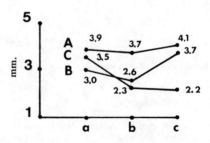

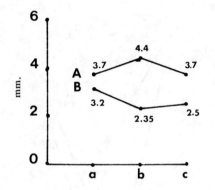

Figure 2.10

Finger Pulse Volume During Breathing Practices. (Wenger and Bagchi)[5]

A = Kapalabhati (Skull-Shining)
B = Hyperventilation after Kapalabhati

a = Pre-Exercise Period
b = Exercise Period
c = Post-Exercise Period

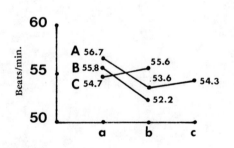

Figure 2.11

Basal Heart Rate. (Dhanaraj)[7]

A = Yoga Group
B = 5BX Group
C = Control Group

a = Initial
b = After 6 wks. Training
c = After 6 wks Detraining

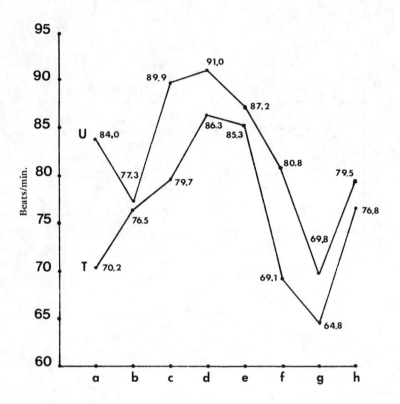

Figure 2.12

Heart Rate during Various Asanas. (Gopal, *et al.*)[8]

T = Trained Subjects
U = Untrained Subjects

a = Inverted Action
b = Shoulder stand
c = Headstand
d = Bridge Posture
e = Half-Spinal Twist
f = Symbol of Yoga
g = Corpse Posture
h = Adamant Posture

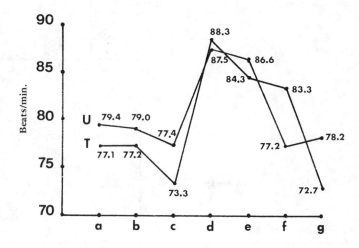

Figure 2.13

ECG Heart Rate during Various Breathing
Patterns. (Gopal, *et al.*)[4]

T = Trained Subjects
U = Untrained Subjects

a = Normal Rhythmic Breathing
b = Rhythmic Inspiration
c = Rhythmic Expiration
d = Deep Inspiration with Locks
e = Deep Expiration with Locks
f = Deep Inspiration without Locks
g = Deep Expiration without Locks

Figure 2.14

Pulse Rate   (Udupa, *et al.*)[9]

a = Initial
b = After 3 mos. of Yoga
c = After 6 mos. of Yoga

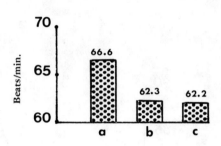

Figure 2.15

Increase in Pulse Rate after Fast Running.
(Udupa, *et al.*)[11]

a = Initial
b = After 3 mos. Training in Yoga
c = After 6 mos. Training in Yoga

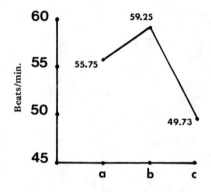

Figure 2.16

Pulse Rate while Standing.   (Udupa, *et al.*)[10]

A = After 3 mos. Practice of Postures
B = Before

a = Sun-Salutation Practiced
b = Sun-Salutation Practiced
c = Headstand and Peacock Practiced
d = Shoulder stand, Fish, and Plow
     Practiced

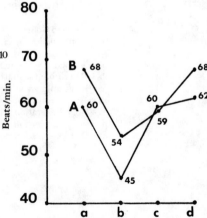

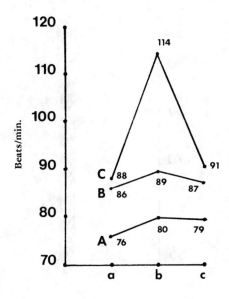

Figure 2.17

Heart Rate during Breathing Practices.
(Wenger and Bagchi)[5]

A = Ujjayi
B = Bhastrika (Bellows)
C = Hyperventilation after Bhastrika

a = Pre-Exercise Period
b = Exercise Period
c = Post-Exercise Period

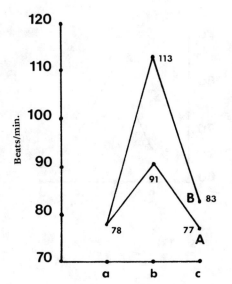

Figure 2.18

Heart Rate during Breathing Practices.
(Wenger and Bagchi)[5]

A = Kapalabhati (Skull-Shining)
B = Hyperventilation after Kapalabhati

a = Pre-Exercise Period
b = Exercise Period
c = Post-Exercise Period

Figure 2.19

Heart Rate during Shoulder
Stand. (Dhanaraj)[7]

a = Basal Value
b = Shoulder stand Value

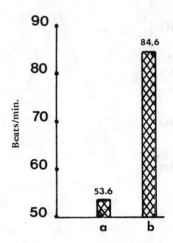

Figure 2.20

Heart Rate with the Body in Various
Positions. (Rao)[2]

a = Horizontal Supine Position
b = Erect Standing Position
c = Headstand Position
d = Horizontal Supine Position

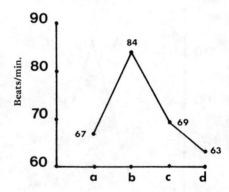

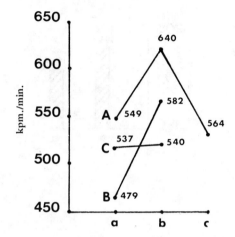

Figure 2.21

PWC$_{130}$ (Dhanaraj)[7]

A = Yoga Group
B = 5BX Group
C = Control Group

a = Initial
b = After 6 wks. Training
c = After 6 wks. Detraining

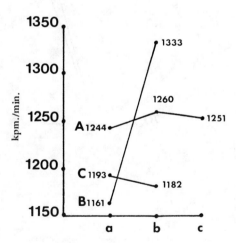

Figure 2.22

PWC$_{170}$ (Dhanaraj)[7]

A = Yoga Group
B = 5BX Group
C = Control Group

a = Initial
b = After 6 wks. Training
c = After 6 wks. Detraining

Figure 2.23

Maximal Heart Rate.
(Dhanaraj)[7]

a = Before
b = After 6 wks. Yoga Training

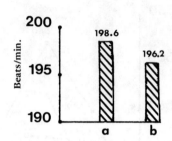

Figure 2.24

Pulse Rate Before and After
Standard Physical Exercise.
(Gopal, *et al.*)[20]

T = Trained Group
U = Untrained Group

a = Before Standard Physical Exercise
b = After Standard Physical Exercise

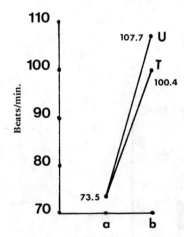

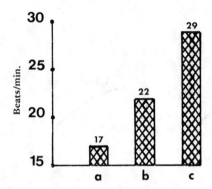

Figure 2.25

Pulse Deceleration after Exercise.
(Dhanaraj)[7]

a = Sitting after Exercise
b = Engaging in Mild Exercise
after Exercise
c = Practicing the Corpse Posture
after Exercise

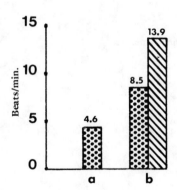

Figure 2.26

Pulse Deceleration after Sitting.
(Dhanaraj)[7]

= Supine Rest
= Corpse Posture

a = Yoga Group before Training
b = After 6 wks. Yoga Training
(is Control Group)

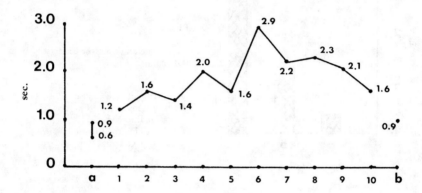

Figure 2.27

Heart Period. (Wenger, *et al.*)[28]

a = Initial Range
b = Just after Heart Slowing Maneuver
1, ..., 10 = Last 10 Heart Periods
during Heart Slowing Maneuver

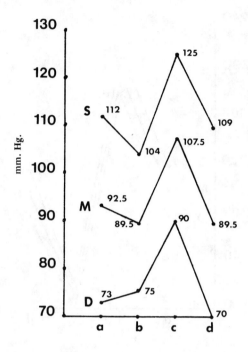

Figure 2.28

Brachial Blood Pressure with Body in
Various Positions. (Rao)[2]

D = Diastolic Blood Pressure
M = Mean Blood Pressure
S = Systolic Blood Pressure

a = Horizontal Supine Position
b = Erect Standing Position
c = Headstand Position
d = Horizontal Supine Position

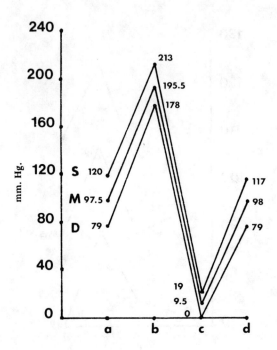

Figure 2.29

Posttibial Blood Pressure with Body
in Various Positions. (Rao)[2]

D = Diastolic Blood Pressure
M = Mean Blood Pressure
S = Systolic Blood Pressure

a = Horizontal Supine Position
b = Erect Standing Position
c = Headstand Position
d = Horizontal Supine Position

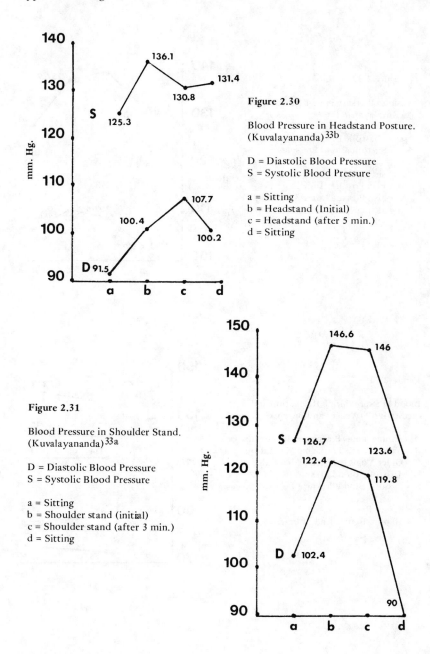

Figure 2.30

Blood Pressure in Headstand Posture.
(Kuvalayananda)[33b]

D = Diastolic Blood Pressure
S = Systolic Blood Pressure

a = Sitting
b = Headstand (Initial)
c = Headstand (after 5 min.)
d = Sitting

Figure 2.31

Blood Pressure in Shoulder Stand.
(Kuvalayananda)[33a]

D = Diastolic Blood Pressure
S = Systolic Blood Pressure

a = Sitting
b = Shoulder stand (initial)
c = Shoulder stand (after 3 min.)
d = Sitting

Figure 2.32

Blood Pressure in Fish Posture.
(Kuvalayananda)[33a]

D = Diastolic Blood Pressure
S = Systolic Blood Pressure

a = Sitting
b = Fish Posture (Initial)
c = Fish Posture (after 3 min.)
d = Sitting

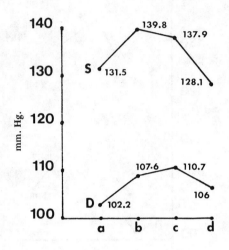

Figure 2.33

Blood Pressure during Relaxation and
Meditation. (Wenger and Bagchi)[5]

A = Young Yogis Practicing Corpse Posture
B = Young Yogis Practicing Meditation
C = Older Yogis Practicing Meditation
D = Diastolic Blood Pressure
S = Systolic Blood Pressure

a = Before Practice
b = 10 min. Before End of Practice

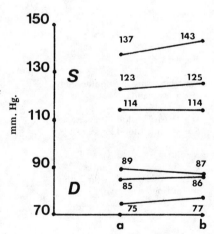

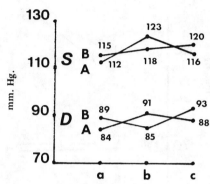

Figure 2.34

Blood Pressure during Breathing Practices.
(Wenger and Bagchi)[5]

A = Kapalabhati (Skull Shining)
B = Hyperventilation after Kapalabhati
D = Diastolic Blood Pressure
S = Systolic Blood Pressure

a = Pre-Exercise Peiod

a = Pre-Exercise Period
b = Exercise Period
c = Post-Exercise Period

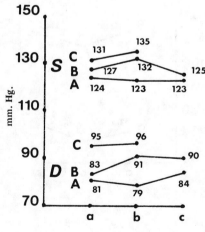

Figure 2.35

Blood Pressure during Breathing Practices.
(Wenger and Bagchi)[5]

A = Ujjayi
B = Bhastrika (Bellows)
C = Hyperventilation after Bhastrika
D = Diastolic Blood Pressure
S = Systolic Blood Pressure

a = Pre-Exercise Period
b = Exercise Period
c = Post-Exercise Period

Figure 2.36

Blood Pressure before and
after Standard Physical
Exercise. (Gopal, *et al.*)[20]

D = Diastolic Blood Pressure
S = Systolic Blood Pressure
T = Trained Subjects
U = Untrained Subjects

a = Before Standard Physical Exercise
b = After Standard Physical Exercise

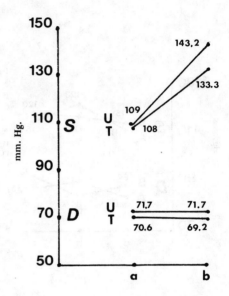

Figure 2.37

Basal Blood Pressure after
Yoga Training. (Udupa, *et al.*)[9]

D = Diastolic Blood Pressure
S = Systolic Blood Pressure

a = Initial
b = After 3 mo. of Yoga
c = After 6 mo. of Yoga

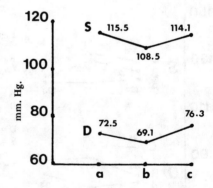

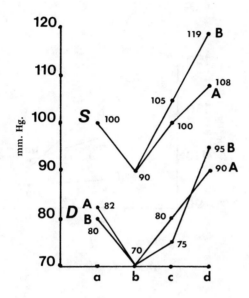

Figure 2.38

Blood Pressure (Standing)
(Udupa, *et al.*)[10]

 A = After 3 mos. Training
B = Initial
D = Diastolic Blood Pressure
S = Systolic Blood Pressure

a = Sun Salutation Practiced
b = Sun Salutation Practiced
c = Headstand and Peacock
    Postures Practiced
d = Shoulder stand, Fish and
    Plow Postures Practiced

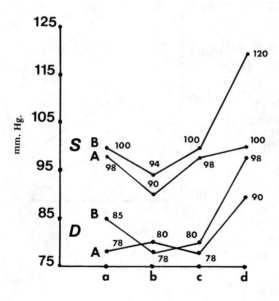

Figure 2.39

Blood Pressure (Sitting)
(Udupa, *et al.*)[10]

A = After 3 mos. Training
B = Initial
D = Diastolic Blood Pressure
S = Systolic Blood Pressure

a = Sun Salutation Practiced
b = Sun Salutation Practiced
c = Headstand and Peacock
    Postures Practiced
d = Shoulder stand, Fish and
    Plow Postures Practiced

Figure 2.40

Mean Blood Pressure of
Hypertensives after Yoga
Relaxation Training.
(Datey, *et al.*)[39]

A = Subjects not Using Drugs
B = Subjects whose B. P. Adequately
    Controlled by Drugs
C = Subjects whose B. P. not
    Adequately Controlled by
    Drugs

a = Before Yoga Relaxation
    Training
b = After Yoga Relaxation
    Training

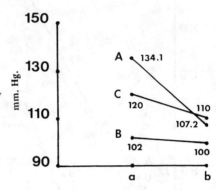

Figure 2.41

Blood Pressure of Hyper-
tensives after Yoga and
Biofeedback Training.
(Patel)[40]

D = Diastolic Blood Pressure
M = Mean Blood Pressure
S = Systolic Blood Pressure

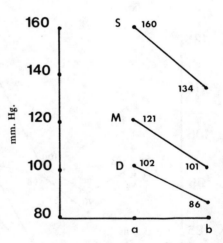

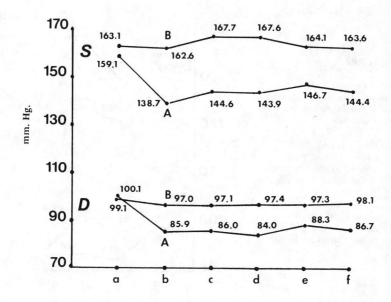

Figure 2.42

Blood Pressure of Hyper-
tensives after Training and
Followup in Yoga Relaxation
and Biofeedback. (Patel)[41]

A = Yoga Relaxation and
        Biofeedback Group
B = Control Group
D = Diastolic Blood Pressure
S = Systolic Blood Pressure

a = Initial
b = End of Yoga Training
c = End of Control Group
        "Training"
d, e, f = 3 mo. Followup
        Intervals

Figure 2.43

Blood Pressure of Hyper-
tensives after Yoga Relaxation
and Biofeedback Training.
(Patel and North)[42]

A = Group A (See Text)
B = Group B (See Text)
D = Diastolic Blood Pressure
S = Systolic Blood Pressure

a = Phase 1, Initial
b = Phase 1, after 6 wks.
c = Phase 2, Initial
d = Phase 2, after 6 wks.

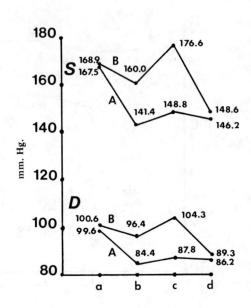

Figure 2.44

Hematocrit. (Dhanaraj)[7]

A = Yoga Group
B = 5BX Group
C = Control Group

a = Initial
b = After 6 wks. Training
c = After 6 wks. Detraining

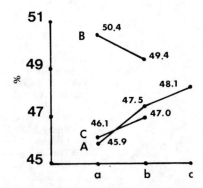

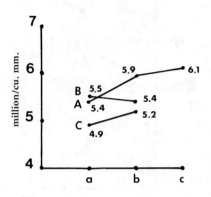

Figure 2.45

Red Blood Cell Count.
(Dhanaraj)[7]

A = Yoga Group
B = 5BX Group
C = Control Group

a = Initial
b = After 6 wks. Training
c = After 6 wks. Detraining

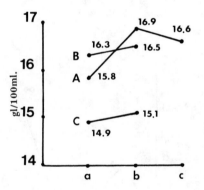

Figure 2.46

Hemoglobin. (Dhanaraj)[7]

A = Yoga Group
B = 5BX Group
C = Control Group

a = Initial
b = After 6 wks. Training
c = After 6 wks. Detraining

Figure 2.47

Total Leucocyte Count.
(Udupa, *et al.*)[10]

A = After 3 mos. Training
B = Initial

a = Sun Salutation Practiced
b = Sun Salutation Practiced
c = Headstand and Peacock
    Postures Practiced
d = Shoulder stand, Fish and
    Plow Postures Practiced

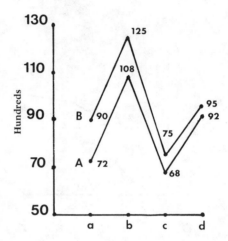

Figure 2.48

Total Serum Protein after
Yoga Training. (Udupa, *et al*)[9]

a = Initial
b = After 3 mo. Training
c = After 6 mo. Training

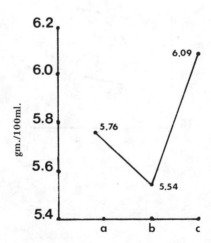

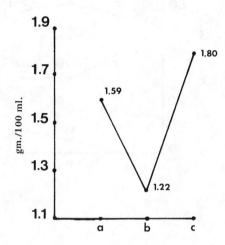

Figure 2.49

Serum Globulin after
Yoga Training.
(Udupa, *et al.*)[9]

a = Initial
b = After 3 mo. Training
c = After 6 mo. Training

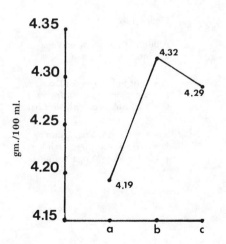

Figure 2.50

Serum Albumin after
Yoga Training.
(Udupa, *et al.*)[9]

a = Initial
b = After 3 mo. Training
c = After 6 mo. Training

Figure 2.51

Total Protein Changes after
Yoga Training. (Gopal, *et al.*)[47]

A = % of Subjects with Decrease
B = % of Subjects with Increase
c = % of Subjects with No Change

a = After 1 mo. Yoga Training
b = After 3 mo. Yoga Training
c = After 6 mo. Yoga Training

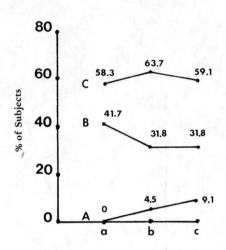

Figure 2.52

Albumin Changes after Yoga
Training. (Gopal, *et al.*)[47]

A = % of Subjects with Decrease
B = % of Subjects with Increase
C = % of Subjects with No Change

a = After 1 mo. Yoga Training
b = After 3 mo. Yoga Training
c = After 6 mo. Yoga Training

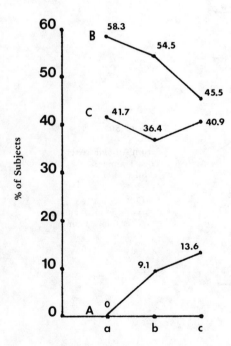

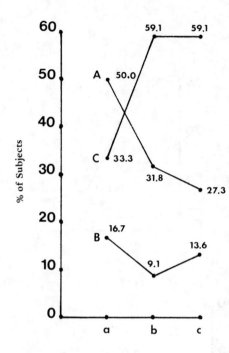

Figure 2.53

Globulin Changes after Yoga Training. (Copal, *et al.*)[47]

A = % of Subjects with Decrease
B = % of Subjects with Increase
C = % of Subjects with No Change

a = After 1 mo. Yoga Training
b = After 3 mo. Yoga Training
c = After 6 mo. Yoga Training

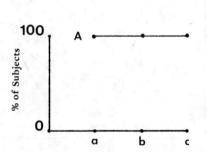

Figure 2.54

Creatinine, Urea Changes after Yoga Training. (Gopal, *et al.*)[47]

A = % of Subjects with No Change

a = After 1 mo. Yoga Training
b = After 3 mo. Yoga Training
c = After 6 mo. Yoga Training

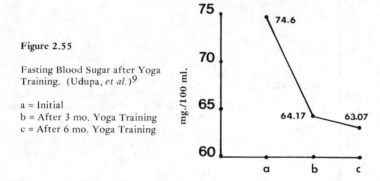

Figure 2.55

Fasting Blood Sugar after Yoga
Training. (Udupa, *et al.*)[9]

a = Initial
b = After 3 mo. Yoga Training
c = After 6 mo. Yoga Training

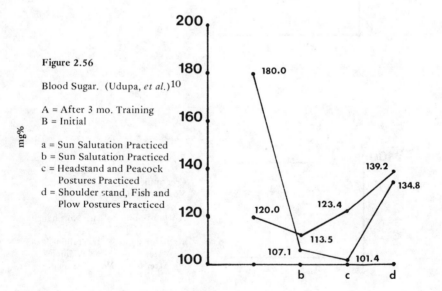

Figure 2.56

Blood Sugar. (Udupa, *et al.*)[10]

A = After 3 mo. Training
B = Initial

a = Sun Salutation Practiced
b = Sun Salutation Practiced
c = Headstand and Peacock
      Postures Practiced
d = Shoulder stand, Fish and
      Plow Postures Practiced

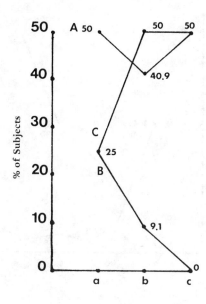

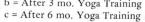

Figure 2.57

Blood Sugar Changes after Yoga Training. (Gopal, *et al.*)[47]

A = % of Subjects with Decrease
B = % of Subjects with Increase
C = % of Subjects with No Change

a = After 1 mo. Yoga Training
b = After 3 mo. Yoga Training
c = After 6 mo. Yoga Training

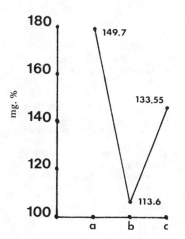

Figure 2.58

Serum Cholesterol after Yoga Training. (Udupa, *et al.*)[9]

a = Initial
b = After 3 mo. Yoga Training
c = After 6 mo. Yoga Training

Figure 2.59

Plasma Cholesterol. (Udupa,
et al.)[10]

A = After 3 mo. Training
B = Initial

a = Sun Salutation Practiced
b = Sun Salutation Practiced
c = Headstand and Peacock
    Postures Practiced
d = Shoulder stand, Fish and
    Plow Postures Practiced

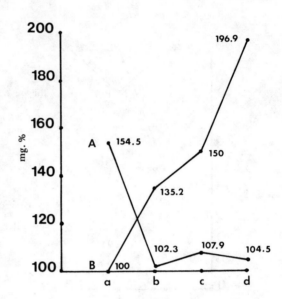

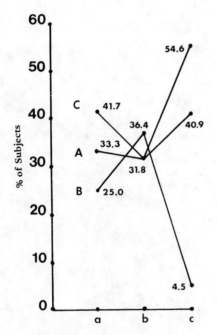

Figure 2.60

Cholesterol Changes after Yoga
Training. (Gopal, *et al.*)[47]

A = % of Subjects with Decrease
B = % of Subjects with Increase
C = % of Subjects with No Change

a = After 1 mo. Yoga Training
b = After 3 mo. Yoga Training
c = After 6 mo. Yoga Training

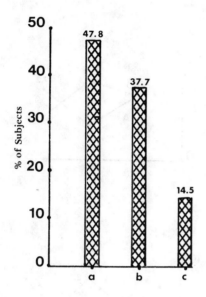

Figure 3.1

Nostril Dominance.
(Bhole and Karambelkar)[2]

a = Left Nostril Dominant
b = Right Nostril Dominant
c = Left and Right Nostrils Equal

Figure 3.2

Nostril Dominance and Placement of
Crutch under Arm. (Bhole and
Karambelkar)[2]

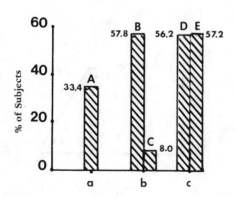

A = Left Nostril Dominant when
  Crutch under Right Arm
B = Right Nostril Dominant when
  Crutch under Right Arm
C = Right Nostril Dominant when
  Crutch under Left Arm
D = Left Nostril Dominant when
  Crutch under Right Arm
E = Right Nostril Dominant when
  Crutch under Left Arm

a = Initial Right Nostril Dominance
b = Initial Left Nostril Dominance
c = Initial Equal Nostril Dominance

Figure 3.3

Differential Minute Ventilation.
(Rao and Potdar)[3]

A = Right Nasal Ventilation
B = Left Nasal Ventilation

a = Normal in Sitting
b = Crutch under Right Arm
c = Crutch under Left Arm

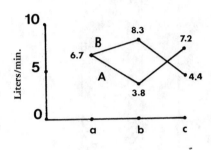

Figure 3.4

Differential Minute Ventilation.
(Rao and Potdar)[3]

A = Right Nasal Ventilation
B = Left Nasal Ventilation

a = Normal in Supine
b = Right Lateral Position
c = Left Lateral Position

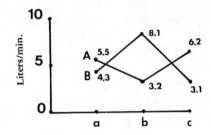

Figure 3.5

Basal Breath Rate after Yoga
Training. (Udupa, *et al.*)[4]

a = Initial
b = After 3 mo. Yoga Training
c = After 6 mo. Yoga Training

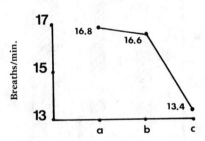

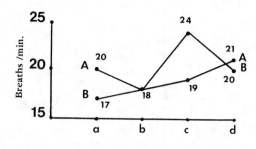

Figure 3.6

Breath Rate (Standing)
(Udupa, *et al.*)[5]

A = After 3 mo. Training
B = Initial

a = Sun Salutation Practiced
b = Sun Salutation Practiced
c = Headstand, Peacock
    Practiced
d = Shoulder stand, Fish, Plow
    Practiced

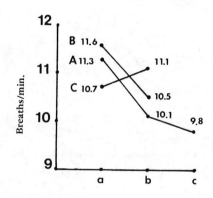

Figure 3.7

Basal Breath Rate
(Dhanaraj)[6]

A = Yoga Group
B = 5BX Group
C = Control Group

a = Initial
b = After 6 wk. Training
c = After 6 wk. Detraining

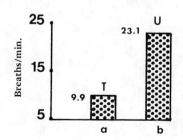

Figure 3.8

Breath Rate in Normal Rhythmic
Breathing. (Gopal, *et al.*)[8]

T = Trained Subjects
U = Untrained Subjects

Figure 3.9

Breath Rate before and after
Standard Physical Exercises.
(Gopal, *et al.*)[20]

T = Trained Subjects
U = Untrained Subjects

a = Before Standard Physical Exercises
b = After Standard Physical Exercises

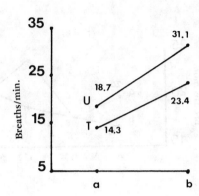

Figure 3.10

Breath Rate during Yoga Postures
(Gopal, *et al.*)[8]

T = Trained Subjects
U = Untrained Subjects

a = Inverted Posture
b = Shoulder stand Posture
c = Headstand Posture
d = Bridge Posture
e = Half-Spinal Twist Posture
f = Symbol of Yoga
g = Corpse Posture
h = Adamant Posture

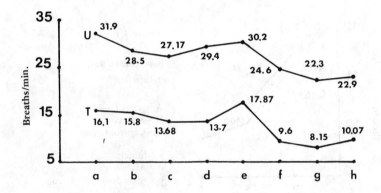

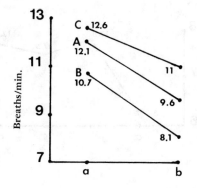

Figure 3.11

Breath Rate. (Dhanaraj)[11]

A = Subjects Practicing Yoga Relaxation
B = Subjects Practicing Meditation
C = Control Subjects in Supine Rest

a = Before Practice
b = After Practice

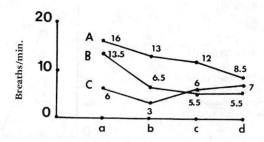

Figure 3.12

Breath Rate. (Wenger and Bagchi)[9]

A = Young Yogis Practicing Corpse Posture
B = Young Yogis Practicing Meditation
C = Older Yogis Practicing Meditation

a = 5 min. Before Practice
b = After 5 min. of Practice
c = Middle of Practice
d = 10 min. before End of Practice

Science Studies Yoga

Figure 3.13

Breath Rate with Body in
Various Positions.(Rao)[12]

a = Horizontal Supine Position
b = Erect Standing Position
c = Headstand Position
d = Horizontal Supine Position

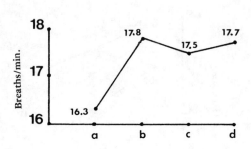

Figure 3.14

Breath Rate. (Miles)[13]

a = Pre-Exercise Period
b = Exercise Period
    (Ujjayi Breathing)
c = Post-Exercise Period

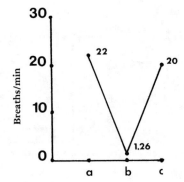

Figure 3.15

Breath Rate during Yoga Breathing
at Low and High Altitudes. (Rao)[14]

A = Yoga Breathing (Ujjayi)
B = Normal Breathing

a = Low Altitude
b = High Altitude

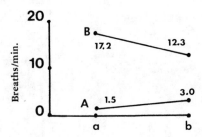

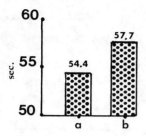

Figure 3.16

Breath Holding Time.
(Gopal, *et al.*)[20]

a = Trained Subjects
b = Untrained Subjects

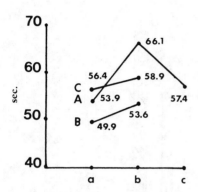

Figure 3.17

Breath Holding Time. (Dhanaraj)[21]

A = Yoga Group
B = 5BX Group
C = Control Group

a = Initial
b = After 6 wk. Training
c = After 6 wk. Detraining

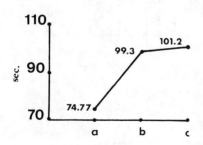

Figure 3.18

Breath Holding Time after Yoga
Training. (Udupa, *et al.*)[22]

a = Initial
b = After 3 mo. Yoga Training
c = After 6 mo. Yoga Training

Figure 3.19

Breath Holding Time.
(Udupa, *et al.*)[5]

A = After 3 mo. Training
B = Initial

a = Sun Salutation Practiced
b = Sun Salutation Practiced
c = Headstand, Peacock
       Practiced
d = Shoulder stand, Fish,
       Plow Practiced

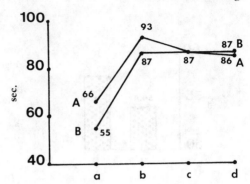

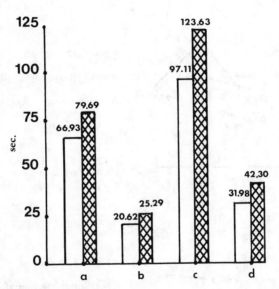

Figure 3.20

Breath Holding Time after Yoga
Training. (Moses)[23]

☐ = Initial
▨ = After 10 wk. Yoga Training

a = After full inhalation
b = After full exhalation
c = After full inhalation preceded
       by Hyperventilation
d = After normal inhalation

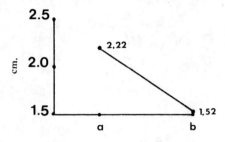

Figure 3.21

Respiratory Amplitude.
(Gopal, *et al.*)[24]

a = Trained Subjects
b = Untrained Subjects

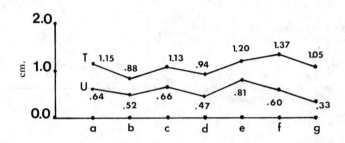

Figure 3.22

Respiratory Amplitude during
Yoga Postures. (Gopal, *et al.*)[25]

T = Trained Subjects
U = Untrained Subjects

a = Inverted Posture
b = Shoulder stand Posture
c = Headstand Posture
d = Bridge Posture
e = Half-Spinal Twist Posture
f = Symbol of Yoga
g = Corpse Posture

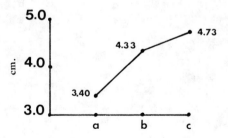

Figure 3.23

Chest Expansion after Yoga
Training. (Udupa, *et al.*)[27]

a = Initial
b = After 3 mo. Yoga Training
c = After 6 mo. Yoga Training

Figure 3.24

Chest Expansion. (Dhanaraj)[28]

A = Yoga Group
B = 5BX Group
C = Control Group

a = Initial
b = After 6 wk. Training
c = After 6 wk. Detraining

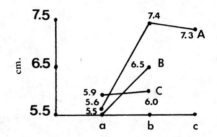

Figure 3.25

Chest Measurement Changes.
(Gopal, *et al.*)[29]

A = Increase over Normal after
     Full Inspiration
B = Decrease over Normal after
     Full Expiration

a = Without Yoga Locks
b = With Yoga Locks

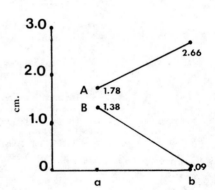

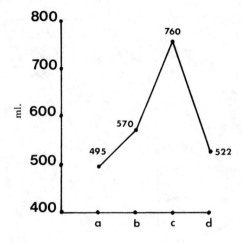

Figure 3.26

Tidal Volume with Body in
Various Positions. (Rao)[30]

a = Horizontal Supine Position
b = Erect Standing Position
c = Headstand Position
d = Horizontal Supine Position

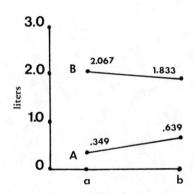

Figure 3.27

Tidal Volume during Yoga
Breathing at Low and High
Altitudes. (Rao)[31]

A = Normal Breathing
B = Yoga Breathing (Ujjayi)

a = Low Altitude
b = High Altitude

Figure 3.28

Tidal Volume during Yoga Relaxation
and Meditation. (Dhanaraj)[32]

A = Subjects Practicing Corpse Posture
B = Subjects Practicing Meditation
C = Control Subjects in Supine Rest

a = Before the Practice
b = After the Practice

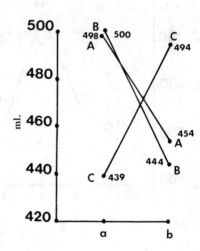

Figure 3.29

Tidal Volume. (Gopal, *et al.*)[33]

a = Trained Subjects
b = Untrained Subjects

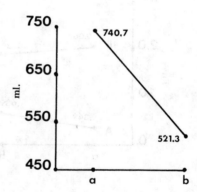

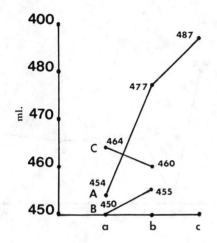

Figure 3.30

Basal Tidal Volume. (Dhanaraj)[34]

A = Yoga Group
B = 5BX Group
C = Control Group

a = Initial
b = After 6 wk. Training
c = After 6 wk. Detraining

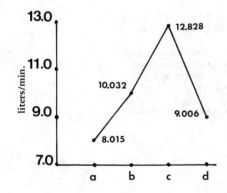

Figure 3.31

Minute Ventilation with Body
in Various Positions. (Rao)[35]

a = Horizontal Supine Position
b = Erect Standing Position
c = Headstand Position
d = Horizontal Supine Position

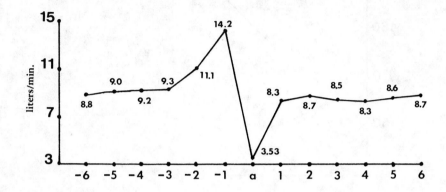

Figure 3.32

Minute Ventilation in a Yoga
Breathing Practice. (Miles)[36]

-6 . . . . -1 = Minutes before
        Yoga Breathing Practice
a = Yoga Breathing Practice
        (Ujjayi)
1 . . . . 6 = Minutes after
        Yoga Breathing Practice

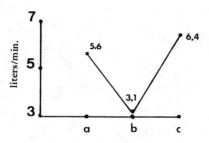

Figure 3.33

Minute Ventilation in a Yoga
Breathing Practice. (Rao)[37]

a = Before Yoga Breathing Practice
b = Yoga Breathing Practice
     (Ujjayi)
c = After Yoga Breathing Practice

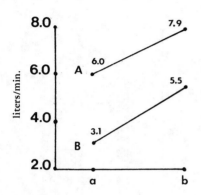

Figure 3.34

Minute Ventilation during Yoga
Breathing at Low and High
Altitudes. (Rao)[37]

A = Normal Breathing
B = Yoga Breathing (Ujjayi)

a = Low Altitude
b = High Altitude

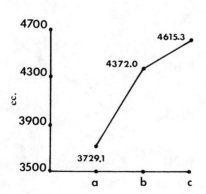

Figure 3.35

Vital Capacity after Yoga
Training. (Udupa, *et al.*)[38]

a = Initial
b = After 3 mo. of Yoga Training
c = After 6 mo. of Yoga Training

Figure 3.36

Vital Capacity. (Dhanaraj)[39]

A = Yoga Group
B = 5BX Group
C = Control Group

a = Initial
b = After 6 wk. Training
c = After 5 wk. Detraining

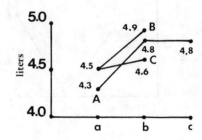

Figure 3.37

Vital Capacity. (Gopal, *et al.*)[40]

a = Trained Subjects
b = Untrained Subjects

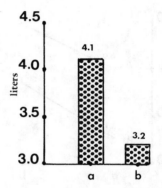

Figure 3.38

Vital Capacity. (Moses)[41]

A = Control Group
B = Yoga Group

a = Initial
b = After 10 wk. Physical
   Education Classes
   (Control) or Yoga
   Class (Yoga)

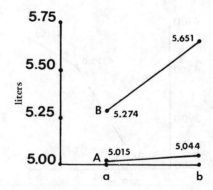

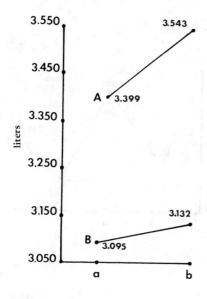

Figure 3.39

Vital Capacity. (Bhole, *et al.*)[42]

A = Yoga Group
B = Control Group

a = Before 3 wk. Experimental
     Period
b = After 3 wk. Experimental
     Period

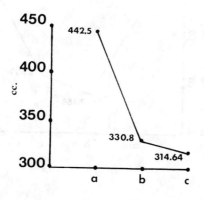

Figure 3.40

Fall in Vital Capacity
after Fast Running.
(Udupa, *et al.*)[43]

a = Initial
b = After 3 mo. Training
     in Yoga
c = After 6 mo. Training
     in Yoga

Figure 3.41

Vital Capacity with Body
in Various Positions. (Rao)[44]

a = Horizontal Supine Position
b = Erect Standing Position
c = Headstand Position
d = Horizontal Supine Position

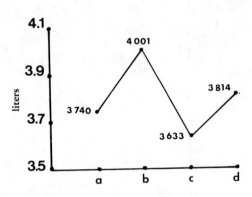

Figure 3.42

Inspiratory Capacity with
Body in Various Positions.
(Rao)[44]

a = Horizontal Supine Position
b = Erect Standing Position
c = Headstand Position
d = Horizontal Supine Position

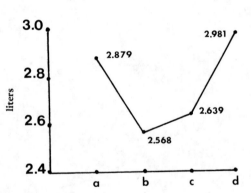

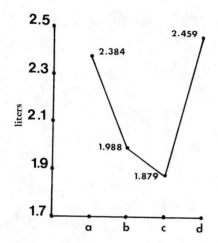

Figure 3.43

Inspiratory Reserve Volume
with Body in Various Positions.
(Rao)[44]

a = Horizontal Supine Position
b = Erect Standing Position
c = Headstand Position
d = Horizontal Supine Position

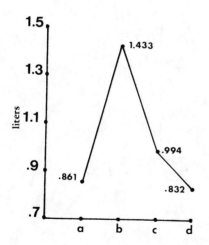

Figure 3.44

Expiratory Reserve Volume
with Body in Various Positions.
(Rao)[44]

a = Horizontal Supine Position
b = Erect Standing Position
c = Headstand Position
d = Horizontal Supine Position

Figure 3.45

Residual Volume with Body in
Various Positions. (Rao)[44]

a = Horizontal Supine Position
b = Erect Standing Position
c = Headstand Position
d = Horizontal Supine Position

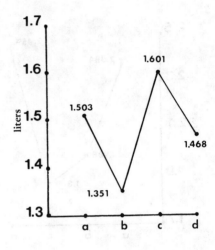

Figure 3.46

Functional Reserve Capacity with
Body in Various Positions. (Rao)[44]

a = Horizontal Supine Position
b = Erect Standing Position
c = Headstand Position
d = Horizontal Supine Position

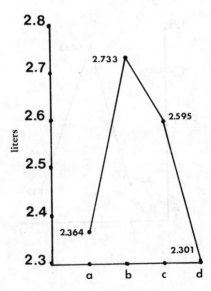

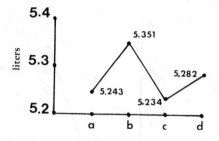

Figure 3.47

Total Lung Capacity with Body in Various Positions. (Rao)[44]

a = Horizontal Supine Position
b = Erect Standing Position
c = Headstand Position
d = Horizontal Supine Position

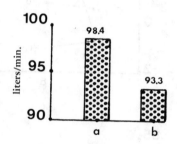

Figure 3.48

Maximum Breathing Capacity. (Gopal, *et al.*)[46]

a = Trained Subjects
b = Untrained Subjects

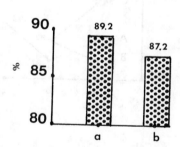

Figure 3.49

Forced Vital Capacity (First Minute). (Gopal, *et al.*)[46]

a = Trained Subjects
b = Untrained Subjects

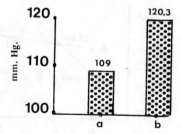

Figure 3.50

Maximum Expiratory Pressure. (Gopal, *et al.*)[46]

a = Trained Subjects
b = Untrained Subjects

Figure 3.51

Basal Metabolic Rate.
(Dhanaraj)[47]

A = Yoga Group
B = 5BX Group
C = Control Group

a = Initial
b = After 6 wk. Training
c = After 6 wk. Detraining

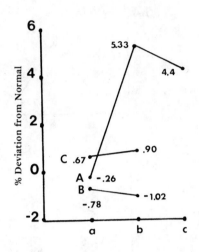

Figure 3.52

Respiratory Quotient.
(Dhanaraj)[47]

A = Yoga Group
B = 5BX Group
C = Control Group

a = Initial
b = After 6 wk. Training
c = After 6 wk. Detraining

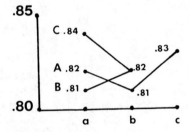

Figure 3.53

Basal Metabolic Rate after Training
in Shoulder stand and Plow Postures.
(Rangan)[48]

A = Control Group
B = Yoga Group

a = Initial
b = After 6 wk. Training

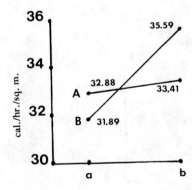

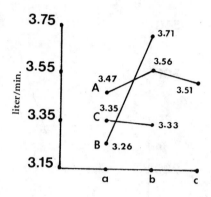

Figure 3.54

Maximum Oxygen Consumption. (Dhanaraj)[47]

A = Yoga Group
B = 5BX Group
C = Control Group

a = Initial
b = After 6 wk. Training
c = After 6 wk. Detraining

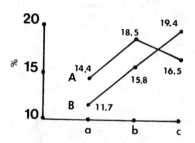

Figure 3.55

Efficiency of Oxygen

Efficiency of Oxygen Utilization. (Salgar, *et al.*)[49]

A = At Low Exercise Level
B = At High Exercise Level

a = Non-Exercise Group
b = Yoga Exercise (Lotus Posture) Group
c = Conventional Exercise Group

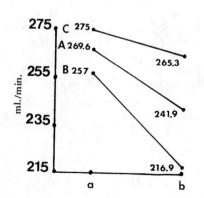

Figure 3.56

Oxygen Consumption. (Dhanaraj)[50]

A = Subjects Practicing Corpse Posture
B = Subjects Practicing Meditation
C = Control Subjects in Supine Rest

a = Before Practice
b = After Practice

Figure 3.57

Oxygen Consumption with
Body in Various Positions.
(Rao)[52]

a = Horizontal Supine Position
b = Erect Standing Position
c = Headstand Position

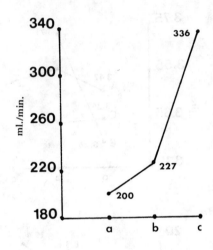

Figure 3.58

Oxygen Consumption during
Various Breathing Practices.
(Miles)[54]

A = Ujjayi
B = Bhastrika (Bellows)
C = Kapalabhati (Skull-Shining)

a = Pre-Exercise Period
b = Exercise Period, First Half
c = Exercise Period, Second
Half
d = Post-Exercise Period, First
5 min.
e = Post-Exercise Period,
Second 5 min.

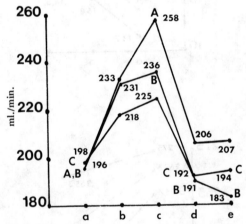

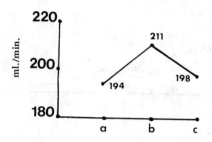

Figure 3.59

Oxygen Consumption during a Yoga Breathing Practice. (Rao)[55]

a = Pre-Exercise Period
b = Yoga Breathing (Ujjayi) Period
c = Post-Exercise Period

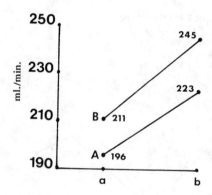

Figure 3.60

Oxygen Consumption during Yoga Breathing at Low and High Altitudes. (Rao)[55]

A = Normal Breathing
B = Yoga Breathing (Ujjayi)

a = Low Altitude
b = High Altitude

Figure 3.61

CO_2 Elimination and O_2 Absorption. (Kuvalayananda)[57]

A = CO_2 Elimination
B = O_2 Absorption

The Count of Time for Inhalation: Retention: Exhalation is
a = 7:0:7
b = 7:0:14
c = 7:7:14
d = 7:0:21
e = 7:14:14
f = 7:0:28

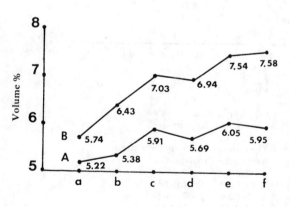

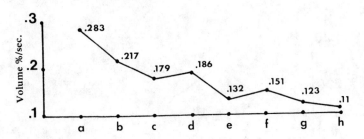

Figure 3.62

CO_2 Elimination Per Second.
(Swami Kuvalayananda)[57]

The Count of Time for Inhalation:
Retention: Exhalation is
a = 7:0:7   e = 7:14:14
b = 7:0:14   f = 7:0:28
c = 7:7:14   g = 7:28:14
d = 7:0:21   h = 7:0:42

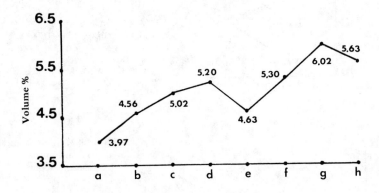

Figure 3.63

CO_2 Elimination.
(Swami Kuvalayananda)[57]

The Count of Time for Inhalation:
Retention: Exhalation is
a = 7:0:7   e = 7:14:14
b = 7:0:14   f = 7:0:28
c = 7:7:14   g = 7:28:14
d = 7:0:21   h = 7:0:42

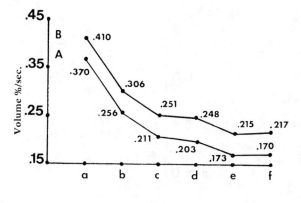

Figure 3.64

CO_2 Elimination and O_2 Absorption, Per Second. (Swami Kuvalayananda)[57]

A = CO_2 Elimination
B = O_2 Absorption

The Count of Time for Inhalation: Retention: Exhalation is
a = 7:0:7
b = 7:0:14
c = 7:7:14
d = 7:0:21
e = 7:14:14
f = 7:0:28
g = 7:28:14
h = 7:0:42

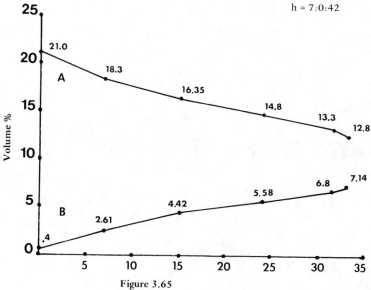

Figure 3.65

Atmospheric Gas Analysis of Subject during a Confinement Experiment. (Gibbons)[59]

A = O_2 Concentration
B = CO_2 Concentration

Figure 4.1

Thyroxine. (Dhanaraj)[1]

A = Yoga Group
B = 5BX Group
C = Control Group

a = Initial
b = After 6 wk. Training
c = After 6 wk. Detraining

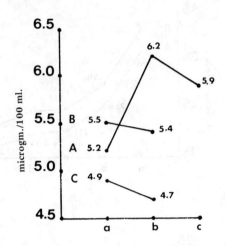

Figure 4.2

Urinary Catecholamines
(VMA) after Yoga
Training (Udupa, *et al.*)[2]

a = Initial
b = After 3 mo. Yoga Training
c = After 6 mo. Yoga Training

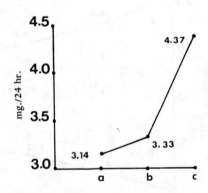

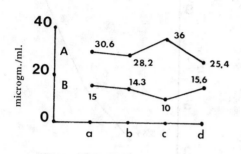

Figure 4.3

Plasma Catecholamines.
(Udupa, *et al.*)[3]

A = After 3 mo. Training
B = Initial

a = Sun Salutation Practiced
b = Sun Salutation Practiced
c = Headstand, Peacock
      Practiced
d = Shoulder stand, Fish,
      Plow Practiced

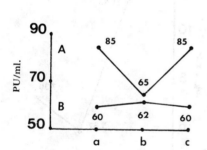

Figure 4.4

Blood Histaminase.
(Udupa, *et al.*)[3]

A = After 3 mo. Training
B = Initial

a = Sun Salutation Practiced
b = Headstand, Peacock
      Practiced
c = Shoulder stand, Fish,
      Plow Practiced

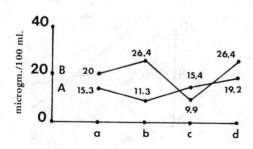

Figure 4.5

Plasma Cortisol.
(Udupa, *et al.*)[3]

A = After 3 mo. Training
B = Initial

a = Sun Salutation Practiced
b = Sun Salutation Practiced
c = Headstand, Peacock
      Practiced
d = Shoulder stand, Fish
      Plow Practiced

Figure 4.6

Urinary 17-Hydroxysteroids
after Yoga Training. (Udupa,
et al.)[2]

a = Initial
b = After 3 mo. Training in Yoga
c = After 6 mo. Training in Yoga

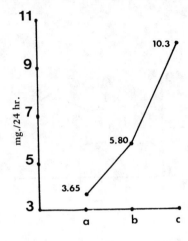

Figure 4.7

Urinary 17-Ketosteroids after
Yoga Training. (Udupa, *et al.*)[2]

a = Initial
b = After 3 mo. Yoga Training
c = After 6 mo. Yoga Training

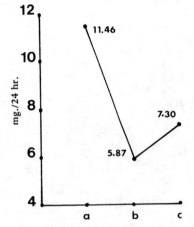

Figure 4.8

Uropepsin Excretion.
(Karambelkar, *et al.*)[5]

A = Yoga Group
B = Control Group

a = Before 3 wk. Test
    Period
b = After 3 wk. Test
    Period

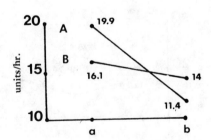

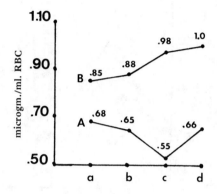

Figure 4.9

Acetylcholine.
(Udupa, *et al.*)[3]

A = After 3 mo. Training
B = Initial

a = Sun Salutation Practiced
b = Sun Salutation Practiced
c = Headstand, Peacock
    Practiced
d = Shoulder stand, Fish,
    Plow Practiced

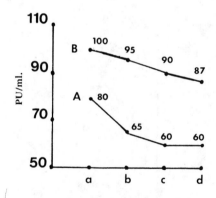

Figure 4.10

Cholinesterase.
(Udupa, *et al.*)[3]

A = After 3 mo. Training
B = Initial

a = Sun salutation Practiced
b = Sun salutation Practiced
c = Headstand, Peacock
    Practiced
d = Shoulder stand, Fish,
    Plow Practiced

Figure 4.11

Plasma Acetycholine after
Yoga Training. (Udupa,
et al.)[7]

a = Initial
b = After 3 mo. Training
     in Yoga
c = After 6 mo. Training
     in Yoga

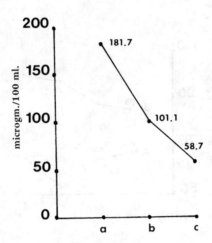

Figure 4.12

Serum Cholinesterase after
Yoga Training. (Udupa, *et al.*)[7]

a = Initial
b = After 3 mo. Training in
     Yoga
c = After 6 mo. Training in
     Yoga

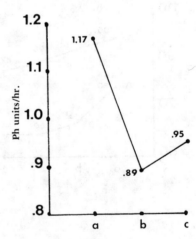

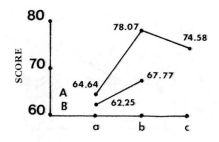

Figure 4.13

Autonomic Balance.
(Gharote)[8]

a = Initial
b = After 2 mo. Training
c = After 2 mo. Detraining

Figure 4.14

Palm-Palm Log Conductance.
(Wenger and Bagchi)[9]

A = Young Yogis Practicing
    Corpse Posture
B = Young Yogis Practicing
    Meditation
C = Older Yogis Practicing
    Meditation.

a = 5 min. before Practice
    Period
b = 5 min. after Start of
    Practice Period
c = Middle of Practice
    Period
d = 10 min. before End
    of Practice Period

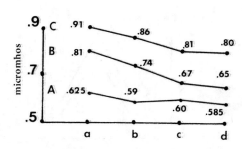

Figure 4.15

Palm-Palm Log Conductance in
Some Yoga Breathing Practices.
(Wenger and Bagchi)[9]

A = Ujjayi
B = Bhastrika (Bellows)
C = Kapalabhati (Skull-Shining)

a = Before Practice Period
b = Practice Period
c = After Practice Period

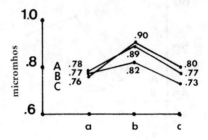

Figure 4.16

Palm-Palm Log Conductance in
Some Breathing Practices.
(Wenger and Bagchi)[9]

A = Kapalabhati (Skull-Shining)
B = Hyperventilation after
    Kapalabhati

a = Pre-Practice Period
b = Practice Period
c = Post-Practice Period

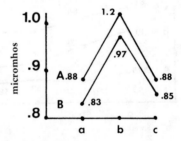

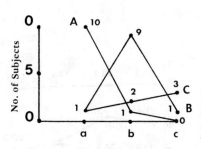

Figure 4.17

Respiratory Movement and EEG Changes. (Timmons, *et al.*)[17]

A = Subjects in Initial Waking
B = Subjects at Onset Stage 1 Sleep
C = Subjects at Onset Stage 2 Sleep

a = Abdominal Amplitude Greater than Thoracic Amplitude
b = Abdominal Amplitude Equal to Thoracic Amplitude
c = Abdominal Amplitude Less than Thoracic Amplitude

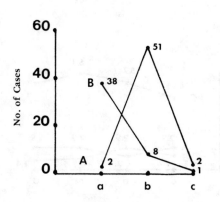

Figure 4.18

Changes in Abdominal Respiration and EEG Transitions. (Timmons, *et al.*)[17]

A = Alpha-Theta Transitions
B = Theta-Alpha Transitions

a = Abdominal Amplitude Increase
b = Abdominal Amplitude Decrease
c = Abdominal Amplitude Unchanged

Figure 5.1

Finger Temperature.
(Wenger and Bagchi)[7]

A = Young Yogis Practicing
    Corpse Posture
B = Young Yogis Practicing
    Meditation
C = Older Yogis Practicing
    Meditation

a = Pre-Practice Period
b = Practice Period, Initial
c = Practice Period, Middle
d= Practice Period, End

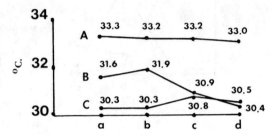

Figure 5.2

Finger Pulse Volume.
(Wenger and Bagchi)[7]

A = Corpse Posture
    (Young Yogis)
B = Meditation
    (Young Yogis)
C = Meditation
    (Older Yogis)

a = Pre-Practice Period
b = Practice Period,
    Initial
c = Practice Period,
    Middle
d = Practice Period,
    End

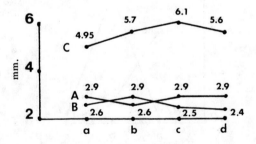

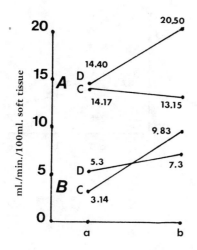

Figure 5.3

Blood Flow.
(Rieckert)[8]

A = Finger Blood Flow
B = Forearm Blood Flow
C = Yoga Meditation Group
D = Autogenic Training
      Group

a = During Rest
b = During Practice of
      Meditation or Autogenic
      Training

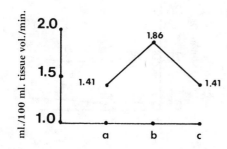

Figure 5.4

Forearm Blood Flow.
(Levander, *et al.*)[9]

a = Pre-Meditation Period
b = Meditation Period
c = Post-Meditation Period

Figure 5.5

Rectal Temperature.
(Wallace, *et al.*)[10]

a = Pre-Meditation Period
b = Meditation Period
c = Post-Meditation
     Period

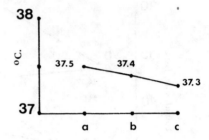

Figure 5.6

Blood Pressure.
(Wallace, *et al.*)[10]

D = Diastolic Blood
     Pressure
M = Mean Blood
     Pressure
S = Systolic Blood
     Pressure

a = Pre-Meditation
     Period
b = Meditation
     Period
c = Post-Meditation
     Period

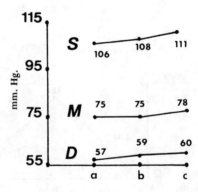

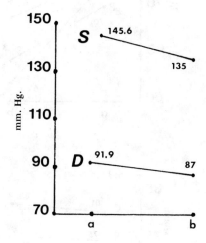

Figure 5.7

Blood Pressure in Hypertensives Who Practiced Meditation. (Benson, *et al.*)[13]

D = Diastolic Blood Pressure
S = Systolic Blood Pressure

a = Before Learning Meditation
b = After 20 wk. Meditation
    Practice

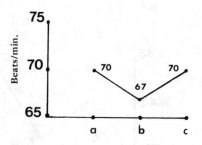

Figure 5.8

Heart Rate.
(Wallace, *et al.*)[10]

a = Pre-Meditation Period
b = Meditation Period
c = Post-Meditation Period

Figure 5.9

Heart Rate. (Dhanaraj)[16]

A = Subjects Practicing Corpse
    Posture
B = Subjects Practicing
    Meditation
C = Control Subjects in
    Supine Rest

a = Before Practice Period
b = After Practice Period

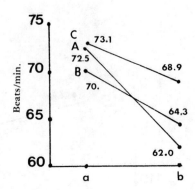

Figure 5.10

Heart Rate. (Wenger
and Bagchi)[7]

A = Young Yogis Practicing
    Corpse Posture
B = Young Yogis Practicing
    Meditation
C = Older Yogis Practicing
    Meditation

a = Pre-Practice Period
b = Practice Period

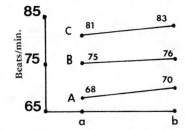

Figure 5.11

PH During Meditation.
(Wallace, *et al.*)[10]

a = Pre-Meditation Period
b = Meditation Period
c = Post-Meditation Period

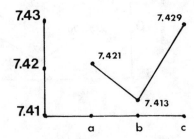

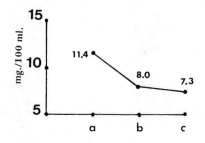

Figure 5.12

Blood Lactate during
Meditation. (Wallace, *et al.*)[10]

a = Pre-Meditation Period
b = Meditation Period
c = Post-Meditation Period

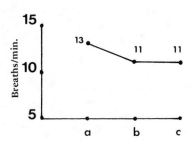

Figure 5.13

Breath Rate during Meditation
(Wallace, *et al.*)[10]

a = Pre-Meditation Period
b = Meditation Period
c = Post-Meditation Period

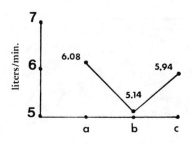

Figure 5.14

Minute Ventilation during
Meditation. (Wallace, *et al.*)[10]

a = Pre-Meditation Period
b = Meditation Period
c = Post-Meditation Period

Figure 5.15

Minute Ventilation during
Meditation. (Wallace)[3]

a . . . . f Denote Time
a, b = Pre-Meditation Period
c, d, e = Meditation Period
f = Post-Meditation Period

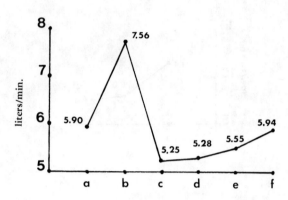

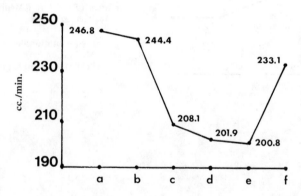

Figure 5.16

Oxygen Consumption during
Meditation. (Wallace)[3]

a . . . . f Denote Time
a, b = Pre-Meditation Period
c, d, e = Meditation Period
f = Post-Meditation Period

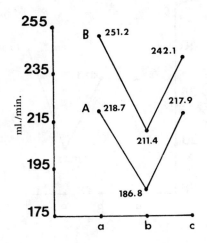

Figure 5.17

Gas Exchange during Meditation. (Wallace, *et al.*)[10]

A = CO_2 Elimination
B = O_2 Consumption

a = Pre-Meditation Period
b = Meditation Period
c = Post-Meditation Period

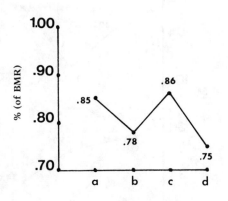

Figure 5.18

Metabolic Rate during Zazen (Sugi, in Hirai)[4]

a, b, c, d = Four Meditating Zen Priests

Figure 5.19

Oxygen Consumption during
Meditation. (Gharote)[36]

a = Basal Metabolic Rate
b = Pre-Meditation Period
c = Meditation Period
d = Post-Meditation Period

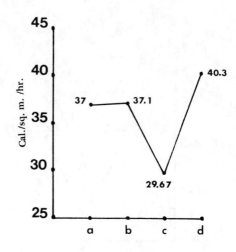

Figure 5.20

Gaseous Partial Pressure during
Meditation. (Wallace, *et al.*)[10]

A = Partial Pressure of Arterial CO_2
B = Partial Pressure of Arterial O_2

a = Pre-Meditation Period
b = Meditation Period
c = Post-Meditation Period

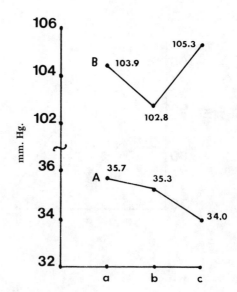

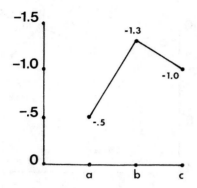

Figure 5.21

Base Excess during Meditation.
(Wallace, *et al.*)[10]

a = Pre-Meditation Period
b = Meditation Period
c = Post-Meditation Period

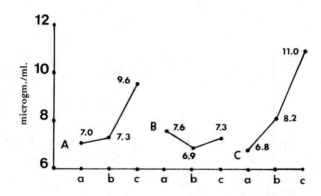

Figure 5.22

Plasma Prolactin.
(Jevning, *et al.*)[41]

A = Long-Term Meditators
B = Control Group before
    Learning Meditation
C = Control Group after 3-4
    mo. Practice of Meditation

a = Pre-Meditation Period
b = Meditation Period (Eyes
    Closed, Gp. B)
c = Post-Meditation Period

Figure 5.23

Plasma Cortisol.
(Jevning, *et al.*)[41]

A = Long-Term Meditators
B = Control Group

a = Pre-Meditation Period
b = Meditation Period (Controls,
    Rest with Eyes Closed)
c = Post-Meditation Period

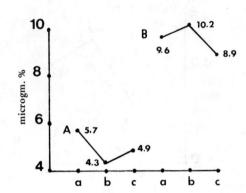

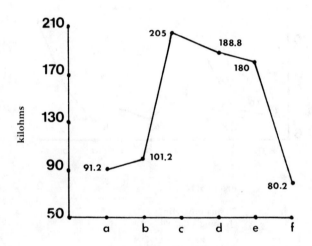

Figure 5.24

Skin Resistance during
Meditation. (Wallace)[3]

a . . . . f Denote Time
a, b = Pre-Meditation Period
c,d,e = Meditation Period
f = Post-Meditation Period

Figure 5.25

Skin Resistance during
Meditation. (Wallace,*et al.*

Skin Resistance during Meditation.
(Wallace, *et al.*)[10]

a = Pre-Meditation Period
b = Meditation Period
c = Post-Meditation Period

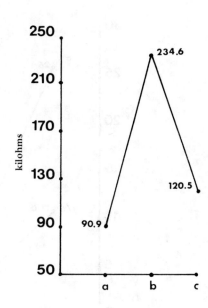

Figure 5.26

Spontaneous GSR.
(Orme-Johnson)[47]

A = Subjects with Meditation
      Experience
B = Control Subjects

a = Rest, Eyes Open
b = Meditation (Rest with
      Eyes Closed for Control
      Subjects)

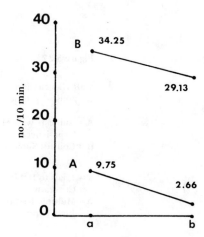

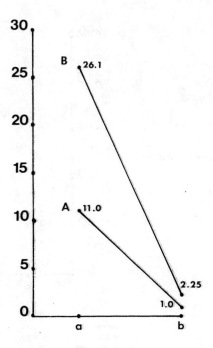

Figure 5.27

GSR Habituation and Multiple
Responses. (Orme-Johnson)[44]

A = Subjects with Meditation
    Experience
B = Control Subjects

a = Trials to Habituation
    Criterion
b = Multiple Responses after
    First Tone

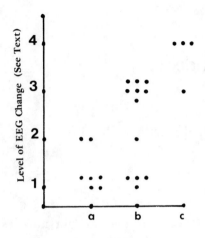

Figure 6.1

EEG Changes in Zazen and
Mental State.
(Kasamatsu and Hirai)[3]

a = Low Mental State
b = Medium Mental State
c = High Mental State

(Mental state of disciples
judged by Zen Master)

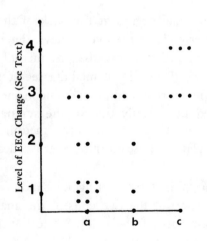

Figure 6.2

EEG Changes in Zazen and
Years of Experience in Zazen.
(Kasamatsu and Hirai)[3]

a = 0-5 yrs. experience
b = 5-20 yrs. experience
c = 20-40 yrs. experience

Appendix C

Glossary of Physiology Terms

ABDOMINAL RECTI, Sing. RECTUS, the two straight muscles of the abdomen crossing it vertically in the front.

ACETYLCHOLINE, a chemical transmitter released at nerve-nerve and nerve-muscle synapses.

ADRENAL GLANDS, a pair of small organs at the back of the abdomen, against the upper ends of the two kidneys. Each adrenal gland consists of two distinct organs: the medulla surrounded by the cortex. The adrenal medulla secretes the catecholamines, epinephrine and norepinephrine; this secretion is increased upon activation of the sympathetic nervous system fibers that innervate the medulla. The adrenal cortex is a gland whose hormones are called corticosteroids.

ANAL SPHINCTERS, the two sphincters, or ringlike bands of muscles, situated an inch apart at the two ends of the anal canal which forms the last part of the colon. The lower and external sphincter constitutes the anus.

ANUS, the posterior opening of the digestive tube.

APNEA, suspension of respiration, partial or entire.

ATMOSPHERIC PRESSURE, pressure exerted by the atmosphere and equal, at sea level, to that of a column of mercury about 760 mm. in height.

AUSCULTATION, listening, as with a stethoscope, for sounds produced in the chest, etc.

AUTONOMIC NERVOUS SYSTEM, that portion of the nervous system which regulates bodily functions other than voluntary movement and conscious sensation, sending efferent fibers to smooth muscles, cardiac muscle and glands. It is comprised of sympathetic and parasympathetic nerves. Many organs receive nerves from both sets and are regulated by the balance of their opposed reactions.

BASAL STATE, a condition of low physical activity suitable for determination of certain normative physiological measurements; usually, the body is in supine rest (not sleep) and several hours have elapsed since food intake and vigorous physical activity.

BICEPS FEMORIS, the large flexor muscle at the back of the thigh.

BRACHIAL, pertaining to the arm.

BLADDER, URINARY, the membranous sac which serves as a reservoir for the urine.

CANALIS CENTRALIS, the central canal which runs throughout the entire length of the spinal cord and is filled with spinal fluid.

CAPILLARY, from the Latin word *capillus*, a hair. A minute blood vessel connecting the smallest ramifications of the arteries with those of the veins.

CECUM, the dilated intestinal pouch into which open the ileum, the colon and the appendix vermiformis.

CEREBROSPINAL NERVOUS SYSTEM, that part of the nervous system which consists of the brain, the spinal cord and the nerves issuing from them.

CERVICAL REGION, that part of the vertebral column covering the neck.

CHOLESTEROL, a fat-like substance in most tissues; blood contains about .2%. It is the main component of deposits in the lining of arteries associated with arteriosclerosis,

heart attack and stroke and the amount of blood cholesterol usually increases with these conditions.

CHOLINESTERASE, a substance which hydrolyzes acetylcholine.

CIRCULATORY SYSTEM, the system consisting of organs
responsible for the circulation of the blood; the organs
are the heart, the arteries, the veins, and the capillaries.

COLON, the portion of the large intestine between the cecum and
the rectum; composed of ascending, transverse and descending sections.

CORTICOSTEROIDS, hormones secreted by the adrenal cortex;
the three physiologically significant ones are corticosterone,
hydrocortisone or cortisol, and aldosterone.

CORTICOSTERONE, a hormone secreted by the adrenal cortex.

CORTISOL, a hormone secreted by the adrenal cortex.

CRANIAL NERVES, the twelve pairs of nerves issuing from the
cranium, or brain.

DIAPHRAGM, the big dome-like muscle that forms the floor of
the thorax, partitioning it from the abdomen.

DIASTOLIC BLOOD PRESSURE, the lowest level of arterial
blood pressure.

ECG, electrocardiogram.   A graphical record of the electrical
current produced by activity of the heart muscle.   The
normal ECG shows upward and downward deflections,
the result of atrial and ventricular activity.   The first upward
deflection, P, is due to contraction of the atria; the other
deflections, Q, R, S, and T, are all due to the action of the
ventricles.

EEG, electroencephalogram.   A graphical record of the electric
currents, developed in the cortex by brain action, which
can be picked up from the surface of the scalp by electrode
leads.

EMG, abbreviation for electromyography or electromyogram.
Electromyography is the study of action potentials, or
electrical changes due to activity, produced by muscle.
The ink-written graphical record of amplifications of these

action potentials is the electromyogram.

ENDOCRINE GLAND, also ductless gland or gland of internal secretion; its product, called a hormone, is released directly into the blood stream to act on other parts of the body. It is distinguished from an exocrine gland of which the secretion (e.g., sweat, digestive juice) flows into a duct to be used locally.

EPINEPHRINE, also known as adrenaline, a hormone released by the adrenal medulla. It increases cardiac output, stimulates the heart muscle, increases the heart rate, elevates blood pressure, elevates blood sugar level.

ESOPHAGUS, the musculo-membranous canal extending from the pharynx to the stomach; in man it is about nine inches long, and passes down the neck between the trachea and the spinal column.

FUNCTIONAL RESERVE CAPACITY, a measure of individual respiratory functioning; the expiratory reserve volume plus the residual volume.

GASTROCNEMIUS, the prominent calf muscle, which extends the foot, flexes the leg, etc.

GLAND, a secreting organ.

GLUTEUS MAXIMUS, the large muscle of the rump.

Hg, abbreviation for the element mercury.

HISTAMINASE, an enzyme with the power of inactivating histamine.

HISTAMINE, a substance which is a powerful dilator of the capillaries and a stimulator of gastric secretion; thought to play a role in allergic reactions.

HORMONE, an internal secretion produced by an endocrine gland and carried by the blood stream to other parts of the body where it has a specific physiological effect.

HYDROXYSTERIOD, a class of hormones produced by the adrenal cortex.

HYPOTHALAMUS, a region of the brain in the floor of the front part of the brain between the cerebral hemispheres.

It is connected by nerve fibers with most other parts of the nervous system. It is the link between the central and autonomic nervous systems and between the nervous system and the endocrine glands. It is involved in visceral controls, emotions, and moods.

INSPIRATORY CAPACITY, the amount of air that can be drawn into the lungs at the end of normal expiration; it averages about 3500 ml.

INSPIRATORY RESERVE VOLUME, the difference between the lung volume at the end of a maximal inspiration and at the end of a normal inspiration; it averages about 3000 ml.

JUGULAR NOTCH, the depression below the throat and between the two collar bones.

KETOSTEROID, a class of hormones produced by the adrenal cortex.

KIDNEYS, the two organs concerned with urine formation.

KPM., abbreviation for kilopond meter (unit of physical work measurement, based on kilopond which is the force acting on one kilogram of mass at the normal acceleration of gravity).

LATISSIMUS DORSI, muscle that covers the lower half of the back; draws the arm downward and backward and rotates it.

LIGAMENT, any tough, fibrous band that connects bones or supports viscera.

LIMBIC SYSTEM, a region of the brain consisting of two rings of medially located cortex along with the amygdaloid, hippocampal and septal nuclei. Along with the hypothalamus it is concerned with sexual behavior and various emotions. It is viewed by some as containing a pleasure center.

LUMBAR, of the part of the back between the lowest pair of ribs and the top of the pelvis; pertaining to the loins.

MEAN BLOOD PRESSURE, diastolic blood pressure plus one-third the pulse pressure.

MEDIASTINUM, the space between the two lungs which contains the heart, major blood vessels, trachea, esophagus, etc.

METABOLISM, the chemical changes by which foods are converted into components of the body or consumed as fuel, the chemical structure of the tissues modified, and waste products are broken down to substances that can be eliminated. The rate of oxygen consumption is used as a measure of metabolic rate.

mg.%, milligram per cent; the number of milligrams of a substance in 100 milliliters of liquid solution.

ml., abbreviation for milliliter.

mm., abbreviation for millimeter.

MUSCLE, the most massive body tissue. The specialized component is the muscle fiber, a long slender cell or agglomeration of cells which becomes shorter and thicker in response to a stimulus. There are three types of muscle. Striated muscle is the flesh or lean meat and is primarily concerned with voluntary movements. Smooth muscle is found in the walls of the digestive and urinary tracts and other hollow organs, and of some blood vessels; smooth muscle is controlled by the autonomic nervous system. Cardiac muscle, the substance of the heart, consists of fibers that contract rhythmically without any nervous impulse, the nerves only modifying the rate of contraction.

NERVE, a bundle of fibers conducting impulses to and from the brain or spinal cord. All nerves are composed from branches of the twelve pairs of cranial nerves and the thirty-one pairs of spinal nerves.

NOREPINEPHRINE, a hormone secreted by the adrenal medulla and also liberated by most sympathetic nerves to act on the smooth muscle or gland innervated by the nerve.

OCCIPITAL REGION, the posterior part of the head.

PANCREAS, a gland situated near the stomach that provides (a) digestive secretion into the small intestine and (b) endocrine secretions of insulin and glucagon, involved with regulation of blood sugar level.

PARASYMPATHETIC NERVOUS SYSTEM, that portion of the autonomic nervous system whose fibers arise from the brain stem and sacral spinal cord.

PARIETAL REGION, that part of the head between the occipital and frontal regions, that forms a part of the top and sides of the head.

PITUITARY GLAND (or hypophysis), an endocrine gland; it consists of two parts, the anterior and posterior lobes. The anterior lobe is a typical endocrine gland, composed of hormone-secreting cells of various kinds, which regulates growth and the activity of several other endocrine glands. The posterior lobe is in effect a modified portion of the nervous system, a protrusion of the hypothalamus, one of whose hormones causes water to be retained by the kidneys.

PLASMA, the clear, fluid portion of blood, freed from blood cells.

PLETHYSMOGRAPH, an instrument for recording variations in the size of various parts of the body, especially such variations as are caused by the circulation of the blood.

POSTTIBIAL, behind the tibia, which is the inner and larger bone of the leg below the knee.

PROLACTIN, a hormone of the anterior pituitary gland; involved in lactation.

PULSE PRESSURE, systolic blood pressure minus diastolic blood pressure.

PWC, physical work capacity; PWC 130, for instance, is the rate of work that a subject can perform when his heart rate is 130 beats per minute.

QUADRICEPS, the great extensor muscle of the front of the thigh.

RESIDUAL VOLUME, the quantity of air, about 1500 ml., that remains in the lungs even after a maximal expiration.

ROLANDIC REGION, motor area of the cerebral cortex.

SERUM, that portion of the blood which remains when fibrinogen is removed from plasma.

SPHINCTER, muscular structure which surrounds a tube or an opening and closes it by contraction.

SPINAL NERVES, thirty-one pairs of nerves that arise from the spinal cord and pass between the vertebrae and from which nerves of the trunk and limbs are derived. At their origin from the spinal cord motor and sensory fibers are in separate roots, motor in front of sensory. Nerves from the upper and lower ends of the spinal cord form networks, the brachial and lumbosacral plexuses, from which branches supply the upper and lower limbs.

STAGE 1 SLEEP, the lightest stage of sleep; characterized by low-voltage, desynchronized EEG activity and sometimes by low-voltage, regular 4-6 Hz. activity as well.

STAGE 2 SLEEP, pattern of sleep following stage 1 sleep after a few seconds or minutes; the EEG is characterized by frequent 13-15 Hz. spindle-shaped tracings, known as sleep spindles, and by certain high-voltage spikes known as K-complexes. In stages 3 and 4 of sleep, high-voltage delta waves appear and then become predominant in the EEG.

STATISTICALLY SIGNIFICANT, occurring by chance only rarely. When a statistic is calculated from data derived from a sample chosen randomly from a population, formulas and tables can be applied to determine the probability p that the statistic for such samples is as extreme as that value calculated for the particular sample data; $p < .01$ means, for example, that the odds are less than 1 in 100 that the data can be explained away as a chance occurrence. If this "p-level" of statistical significance is not stated explicitly, it can (in this treatise) be assumed to be $p < .05$.

SYMPATHETIC NERVOUS SYSTEM, that portion of the autonomic nervous system whose fibers arise from cells in the thoracic and lumbar spinal cord. These cells send fibers to relay stations (ganglia) which form two chains lying in front of the muscles at either side of the backbone. From the sympathetic nerves branches spread throughout the body, most of them accompanying the main arteries.

SYSTOLIC BLOOD PRESSURE, the highest level of arterial blood pressure.

TEMPORAL REGION, region at the temples of the head.

THORAX, the part of the body between the neck and abdomen; the chest.

THYROID GLAND, endocrine gland in the neck near the larynx. Its secretions accelerate the release of energy in the tissues from glucose combustion, thereby increasing breathing and blood circulation to meet the added demand for oxygen; bodily and mental activity are stimulated; body temperature increases. Another secretion facilitates decreased calcium concentration in the blood.

THYROXINE, the most important hormone released by the thyroid gland; contains iodine; has a profound effect on growth.

TIDAL VOLUME, the quantity of air normally inspired with each breath, while at rest; it averages about 500 ml.

TIMED VITAL CAPACITY, the amount of air expired after 1, 2, 3, etc., secs. of maximal forced expiration. Usually the same information is obtained as from the maximal breathing capacity evaluation. The normal person can expire at least 83% of his vital capacity in 1 second.

TOTAL LUNG CAPACITY, a measure of individual respiratory functioning; vital capacity plus residual volume.

UROPEPSIN, a urinary constituent that breaks down protein; believed to be formed in gastric secretions.

VAGUS NERVE, the tenth cranial nerve; it is the most important component of the parasympathetic nervous system. Constriction of the bronchi, slowing of the heart, and stimulation of the digestive organs are some functions of the vagus nerve motor fibers.

VENTILATION, amount of air respired in a unit of time, usually 1 minute; also, called minute ventilation, ventilation volume.

VITAL CAPACITY, the total amount of air that can be moved into or out of the lungs, it is about 4500 ml.

Appendix D

Glossary of Yoga Terms

ABDOMINAL LOCK, *uddiyana-bandha.*

ADAMANT POSTURE, *vajrasana.*

AGNISARA, a hatha yoga practice. While the breath is held after deepest exhalation, the abdomen is alternatively retracted and protracted, each retraction and protraction being maintained for 3-5 seconds, and the process continues until another breath is needed.

ARDHA-MATSYENDRASANA, literally "the half-Lord of the Fishes posture." It is the first in a series of postures that twist the spine. Also called the "half-spinal twist" posture.

ARDHA-SHALABHASANA, half-locust posture.

ASANA, literally "sitting," "position," or "posture." The third of the eight limbs of Raja Yoga, asana emphasizes attainment of a steady and comfortable posture. An asana is a yogic posture which contributes to the steadiness of body and mind and a sense of well-being.

ASTANGA-YOGA, literally "the eight-limbed yoga," referring to the eight steps of classical Raja Yoga as they are explained in Patanjali's *Yoga Sutras.* The eight are *yama* or moral restraints, *niyama* or moral practices, *asana* or posture, *pranayama* or control of the breath and the prana, *pratyahara* or withdrawal and control of the senses, *dharana* or concentration, *dhyana* or meditation, and *samadhi* or superconscious meditation.

BANDHA, literally "lock." A fixed arrangement of contracted muscles.

BELLOWS, *bhastrika.*

BHASTRIKA, literally "the bellows." A breathing exercise where the abdominal muscles and the diaphragm function like a bellows with forced inhalation and exhalation of equal length. "The fast, shallow feature of *kapalabhati* [is] interjected without delays between *ujjayi* cycles. About 20 of the short breaths are taken." (MILES)

BHUJANGASANA, the cobra posture.

BOAT POSTURE, *navasana.*

BOW POSTURE, *dhanurasana.*

BRIDGE POSTURE, *sethubandhasana.*

CHAKRASANA, *wheel posture.*

COBRA POSTURE, *bhujangasana.*

CORPSE POSTURE, *shavasana.*

DAKSHINA-NAULI, the right aspect of nauli, involving isolation of right rectus abdominis.

DHANURASANA, the bow posture.

DHARANA, concentration. The process of bringing the mind, whose natural tendency is to jump from object to object, to voluntary, relaxed attention on a single object. It is the sixth of the eight limbs of yoga described in the *Yoga Sutras.*

DHARMIC ASANA, alternate name for yoga-mudra, or symbol of yoga.

DHYANA, meditation. A steady, natural flow of attention toward one object when the natural tendency of the mind has become to remain withdrawn from the senses and concentrated.

FISH POSTURE, *matsyasana.*

HALASANA, the plow posture.

HALF-SPINAL TWIST, *ardha-matsyendrasana.*

HATHA YOGA, (1) the science of physical culture which developed out of the third limb of Raja Yoga, *asana*, attempts through postures and cleansing exercises to prepare the student for higher practices of yoga. (2) It also denotes the first four limbs of Raja Yoga—*yama, niyama, asana,* and *pranayama* which are known as the external limbs.

HEADSTAND, *shirshasana.*

INVERTED ACTION, *viparitakarani.*

JALANDHARA-BANDHA, the chin-lock, requiring the chin to be closely pressed against the jugular notch or the chest.

JAPA, mental repetition of a mantra which gradually awakens the energy vibrations of which the syllables are the gross representation.

KAPALABHATI, literally, "the shining of the skull, or forehead." A breathing technique where the abdominal muscles and diaphragm make a fast and forceful exhalation followed by a passive inhalation. "A form of shallow, fast, rhythmic breathing, accomplished chiefly by the abdominal muscles. There is no pause introduced between inhalation and exhalation. About two shallow breaths per second for a minute or a little less constitutes a round which is followed by 1 minute of spontaneous breathing. A round of this short-rhythmic breathing is often followed by rather irregular, slow respirations in this two-phase respiratory exercise." (See footnote 13 of Chapter 3.)

KRIYA, see SHAT KRIYAS.

KUMBHAKA, a pause in the breath; the method of retaining the breath in more advanced exercises of pranayama. Retention should not be practiced without the guidance of an experienced and qualified teacher.

LOCK, *bandha.*

LOCUST POSTURE, *shalabhasana.*

MANTRA, (1) a sound, a soothing, helpful sound that vibrates, strengthens and relaxes the nervous system. It is not a religious word. These sounds are found in the deep states of meditation by the great sages. (2) A combination of syllables or words corresponding to a particular energy vibration. The student, when initiated by a qualified teacher, utilizes the mantra as his object for meditation and as he practices over a period of time it gradually leads his meditation deeper and deeper, releasing latent mental and spiritual energies.

MANTRA-YOGA, the set of practices where particular phrases, words and syllables are utilized as objects of meditation to awaken a student's spiritual potential. The essential technique is japa, or mental repetition.

MATSYASANA, the fish posture.

MAYURASANA, the peacock posture.

MUDRA, yogic seal or gesture.

MULA-BANDHA, the anal-contraction or Root Lock, which requires vigorous contraction of the sphincters of the anus.

NADI, a channel in the subtle body for the non-physical vital force called prana; the nadis are in some sense thought to be parallel to the physical nervous system.

NAULI, one of the *shat kriyas*, being an abdominal exercise consisting of the rolling manipulations of the isolated abdominal recti muscles while maintaining the application of *uddiyana bandha.*

NAVASANA, boat posture.

PADMASANA, the lotus posture. A meditative sitting posture recommended for breathing exercises and meditation.

PASHCHIMOTTANASANA, the posterior stretching posture. A head-to-knees posture to stretch the muscles of the back and of the back of the legs.

PATANJALI, the codifier of yoga science; composed the *Yoga Sutras* in the second century B. C.

PEACOCK POSTURE, *mayurasana.*

PLOW POSTURE, *halasana.*

POSTERIOR STRETCHING POSTURE, *paschimottanasana.*

PRANA, the vital life force of any living being which exists in a subtle, non-physical form. It flows through a system of energy channels (*nadis*) which make up the subtle body.

PRATYAHARA, the fifth of the eight limbs of yoga described by Patanjali. The withdrawal and control of the senses which protects the mind from the distractions that come to the senses.

PRANAYAMA, literally, "the control of prana." The science of gradually lengthening and controlling the physical breath in order to gain control over the movements of prana through the subtle body in higher stages of the practice. It is the fourth of the eight steps of yoga described by Patanjali.

RAJA YOGA, literally "the royal path." A recently applied term for the classical system of yoga philosophy and practice codified by the sage Patanjali in the *Yoga Sutras*. Also known as the eight-limbed (*astanga*) yoga because of its eight progressive steps. Sometimes signifies the last four limbs taken together: *pratyahara* or control of the senses, *dharana* or concentration, *dhyana* or meditation, and *samadhi* or superconscious meditation.

SAMADHI, the superconscious state which is the last of the eight limbs of yoga. Samadhi is the subject of the first chapter of the *Yoga Sutras*.

SARVANGASANA, literally "the posture for all limbs." The shoulder stand.

SEAL, *mudra.*

SETHU-BANDHASANA, the bridge posture.

SHALABHASANA, the locust posture.

SHAT KRIYAS, six cleansing processes prescribed in hatha yoga for the purification of the body. They are *neti* for cleansing the nasal passages, *dhauti* for cleansing the stomach, *basti* for cleansing the colon, *trataka* or gazing, *nauli* employed as part of *basti* or for abdominal toning, and *kapalabhati* for cleansing the lungs and air passages.

SHAVASANA, the corpse posture, a supine posture for relaxation.

SHIRSHASANA, the headstand posture.

SHOULDER STAND, *sarvangasana.*

SKULL-SHINING, *kapalabhati.*

SUN-SALUTATION, *suryanamaskar.*

SURYANAMASKAR, the sun salutation; a sequence of 12 body positions. It is not considered to be in the groups of yogic practices but can be considered preliminary to hatha yoga to make the body supple.

SUTRA, literally "a thread." A sutra is an aphorism of the kind used by Indian philosophers to record the progression of the main ideas, the thread of meaning of a philosophical system. Since unnecessary words have been eliminated, a collection of sutras, such as the *Yoga Sutras*, requires commentaries to be understood.

SYMBOL OF YOGA, *yoga mudra; dharmicasana.*

UDDIYANA-BANDHA, the abdominal lock; a lock involving raising of the diaphragm. After a deep exhalation one makes a mock-inhalation, that is, inspiratory movements with glottis closed.

UJJAYI, variety of pranayama characterized by a smooth frictional sound through the throat, due to partial closure of the glottis in breathing. It is "a thoracic type of breathing; abdominal muscles play a passive role . . . a very deep inspiration is taken slowly with the glottis partially closed and the head erect; [while maintaining the chin lock] the breath is held for 40 or more seconds, the head is then raised into the initial position, and slow, deep expiration completes the cycle." (See Reference 13 of Chapter 3.)

USHTRASANA, the camel posture.

VAJRASANA, the pelvic posture, or adamant posture, one version of which involves sitting so the entire body weight rests on the knees in front and the heels and ankles in the rear, with the soles of the feet facing up.

VIPARITAKARANI, inverted action or posture.

VRISCHIKASANA, the scorpion posture.

YOGA, generated from the samskrt root *yuj* which means "to join or apply," yoga means "union" as well as the systematic "application" of certain practices which have effects and benefits tested by many centuries of practitioners. The school of Indian philosophy which, in addition to its philosophical tenets, includes a comprehensive system of practices through which the philosophical "truths" can be tested in actual experience by the student working to perfect himself physically, mentally and spiritually. It is a universal exact science for developing human potential evolved over perhaps five thousand years of self-experimentation by its practitioners. The system was first codified by the sage Patanjali in his *Yoga Sutras* in about the second century B.C.

YOGA DANDA, a small wooden crutch used to modify nostril activity; it is placed under an armpit and is pressed on for some time.

YOGA-MUDRA, the symbol of yoga; a particular posture or gesture.

YOGA-SUTRAS, 196 aphorisms on Raja Yoga, composed by the sage Patanjali at about the date, according to traditional sources, of 200 B.C. It forms the basic outline from which all systems of yoga philosophy and practice claim their origin. It is divided into four main sections or chapters called *padas: Samadhi-pada* concerning superconscious meditation; *Sadhana-pada* concerning spiritual practices, *Vibhuti-pada* concerning attainments, and *Kaivalya-pada* concerning the state of absoluteness (liberation).

ZAZEN, the seated Zen meditation.

Appendix E

Biographical Notes
on Yoga Researchers

The purpose of APPENDIX E is to suggest the background and affiliation of the yoga researchers mentioned in the treatise. It should not be considered to be complete.

B. K. BAGCHI, Ph.D.; University of Michigan.

RUDOLPH M. BALLENTINE, Jr., M.D. (Duke University); Director of the Biofeedback-Meditation and Combined Therapy Programs of the Himalayan Institute; private practitioner of general and psychosomatic medicine in Glenview, Illinois.

JEAN-PAUL BANQUET, M.D.; Stanley Cobb Laboratories for Psychiatric Research, Massachusetts General Hospital and Harvard Medical School, Boston, Massachusetts.

HERBERT BENSON, M.D. (Harvard, 1961); Associate Professor of Medicine, Harvard Medical School, and Program Director, General Clinical Research Center, Thorndike Memorial Laboratory, Boston City Hospital.

M. V. BHOLE, M.D.; Deputy Director of Scientific Research, Kaivalyadhama, India.

ARUN BORDIA, M.D.; Reader in Cardiology, Tagore Medical College and Hospital, Udaipur, India.

G. S. CHHINA, M.A. (Physiology) and Ph.D. (Neurophysiology)

from Punjab University; Department of Physiology, All-India Institute of Medical Sciences, New Delhi, India.

D. P. DALVI, M.D., F.I.C.A.; Department of Cardiology, King Edward Memorial Hospital, Bombay, India.

K. K. DATEY, M.D., F.I.C.A.; Department of Cardiology, King Edward Memorial Hospital, Bombay, India.

S. N. DESHMUKH, M.D., Department of Cardiology, King Edward Memorial Hospital, Bombay, India.

V. H. DHANARAJ, Ph.D. (Physical Education); University of Alberta, Edmonton, Alberta, Canada.

NORM DON, Ph.D.; Union Graduate School, Yellow Springs, Ohio, and Department of Psychiatry, The Pritzker School of Medicine,The University of Chicago.

S. K. GANGULY; Research Assistant, Scientific Research Department, Kaivalyadhama, India.

M. L. GHAROTE, M.A., M.Ed. (Phy. Ed.), D.Y.P.; Assistant Director of Research, Kaivalydhama, India.

K. S. GOPAL, M.Sc.; Biology Department at Jawaharlal Institute of Postgraduate Medical Education and Research, Gorimedu; Ananda Ashram, Pondicherry, India 605006.

M. V. GOVINDASWAMY, M.D.; Director, All-India Institute of Mental Health, Bangalore.

ELMER E. GREEN, Ph.D. (Physics); Research Department, The Menninger Foundation, Topeka, Kansas 66601.

O. P. GUPTA, M.D.; Professor of Pathology, Tagore Medical College and Hospital, Udaipur, India.

JAMES V. HARDT, Ph.D.; Bio-Cyber-nautics Group, Langley Porter Neuropsychiatric Institute, University of California at San Francisco.

TOMIO HIRAI, M.D. (Medical School of University of Tokyo); Assistant Professor of the Faculty of Medicine, Department of Psychiatry, The Tokyo University Hospital; President of the Japanese Society of Psychiatry and Neurology.

J. HOENIG, M.D.; World Health Organization Consultant (1955-56) at The All-India Institute of Mental Health, Bangalore.

R. JEVNING, Ph.D.;   Department of Medicine, University of California at Irvine.

JOE KAMIYA, Ph.D.;   Langley Porter Neuropsychiatric Institute, San Francisco.

P. V. KARAMBELKAR, Ph.D.;   Joint Director of Scientific Research, Kaivalyadhama.

AKIRA KASAMATSU, M.D.;   Professor of the Medical Faculty, Tokyo University.

L. K. KOTHARI, M.Sc., M.A.M.S.;   Reader in Physiology, Tagore Medical College and Hospital, Udaipur, India.

SWAMI KUVALAYNANDA (1883-1966);   Founder (in 1924) and former Research Director, Kaivalyadhama, which includes an ashram, the S.M.Y.M. Samiti Research laboratory, the G. S. College of Yoga and the Gupta Yogic Hospital; research is published quarterly in the journal *Yoga-Mimamsa*; Kaivalyadhama is located at Lonavala, District Poona, India.

V. L. LEVANDER;   Thorndike and Channing Laboratory, Boston City Hospital; Harvard Medical School.

WALTER R. MILES, M.D.;   Department of Psychiatry, Yale University School of Medicine, New Haven, Connecticut.

ROBSON MOSES, D. Ed., University of Oregon.

DAVID W. ORME-JOHNSON, Ph.D.;   Department of Physiology, University of Texas at El Paso, El Paso, Texas.

ROBERT R. PAGANO; Department of Psychology, University of Washington.

C. H. PATEL, M.D.;   11 Upfield, Croydon, CRO 5DR, Surrey, England.

VIJAYENDRA PRATAP, Ph.D.; (Applied Psychology), University of Bombay.   Founder and Director of SKY Foundation, Philadelphia; Former Assistant Director of Yoga Research at Kaivalyadhama.

SWAMI RAMA;   Founder, Himalayan International Institute of Yoga Science and Philosophy, Glenview, Illinois, U.S.A. and Rishikesh, India;   Research Collaboration with The Menninger Foundation.

S. C. B. RANGAN, M.P.E. (1969), Lakshmibai College of Physical Education, Gwalior, India.

H. V. GUNDU RAO, Ph.D.; Department of Biophysics, All-India Institute of Mental Health, Bangalore.

SHANKER RAO, Ph.D.; Department of Physiology, Gandhi Medical College, Hyderabad-DN, A. P., India.

HANS RIECKERT, Ph.D.; Physiologischen Institut der Universitat, Tubingen, Germany.

D. C. SALGAR; Professor of Physiology, Medical College, Aurangabad, Maharashtra State, India.

GARY E. SCHWARTZ, Ph.D.; Department of Psychology and Social Relations, Harvard University.

BALDEV SINGH; Department of Physiology, All-India Institute of Medical Sciences, New Delhi, India.

R. H. SINGH, Ph.D.; Institute of Medical Sciences, Banaras Hindu University, India.

JONATHAN C. SMITH, Ph.D.; Assistant Professor of Psychology, Roosevelt University, Chicago, Illinois.

BEVERLY TIMMONS, Ph.D.; Langley Porter Neuropsychiatric Institute, San Francisco, California 94122.

K. N. UDUPA, M.D. F.R.C.S., F.A.C.S., F.A.M.S.; Institute of Medical Sciences, Banaras Hindu University, India.

ROBERT KEITH WALLACE, Ph.D. (Physiology); Thorndike and Channing Laboratories, Harvard Medical Unit, Boston City Hospital.

M. A. WENGER, Ph.D.; University of California at Los Angeles.

R. C. WHEELER; Thorndike and Channing Laboratory, Boston City Hospital, Harvard Medical School.

ARCHIE F. WILSON, M.D., Ph.D.; Associate Professor of Medicine at the University of California at Irvine, Orange, California 92668.

Index